Abby Ruby Ph.D.

In Sickness and In Health

Exercise Addiction in Endurance Athletics

ISBN: 1453801227
ISBN-13: 9781453801222

Premise

There is a problem in our society whereby the ideal body is often obtained through unhealthy means. Currently, many who adhere to the rigid social norm of what is aesthetically acceptable diet, purge, or exercise to extremes to create the picture-perfect body. Exercise dependence is a growing phenomenon within the field of psychology, yet some who exercise to extremes are hailed as disciplined and celebrated as successful athletes. *In Sickness and In Health* defines exercise addiction as an attitude, a way of approaching exercise, and not a specific "type" of athlete, such as an Ironman athlete, a runner, etc. Instead, any number of athletes can be considered exercise addicts, whether they train for a 3-mile or 300-mile run.

Introduction

In 1977, *Sports Illustrated* proclaimed Eddie Merckx, the world-class cyclist, to be the fittest athlete in the world. John Collins, a naval captain stationed in Hawaii, disagreed. Following a local road race, Collins leaped on stage and challenged all athletes to prove their level of fitness. To find his winner, Collins combined the three toughest athletic events on the island of Oahu and called the result the Ironman Challenge. The daunting course combined the Waikiki Rough Water Swim, the annual bicycle race around Oahu, and the Honolulu Marathon. The distance totaled a 2.4-mile swim, a 112-mile bike ride, and a 26.2-mile run. Reenacted every year since 1978, Ironman is now thirty-two years old, has drawn over five hundred thousand competitors, and has established itself firmly in the world of sport.

One year after the running of the first ever Ironman challenge in 1978, the first article about exercise addiction was published in *Physician and Sports Medicine*. Although the two occurrences have never been aligned in the past, *In Sickness and In Health* seeks to establish whether there is in fact a connection between the growing popularity of Ironman racing and endurance athletics as a whole and exercise addiction. In an effort to understand the potentially excessive and addictive nature of running, biking, swimming, and pushing oneself beyond what one thinks he or she can do, this book will examine the ways in which a particular and rigid (read: thin) social aesthetic creates exercise addiction and the growing popularity of endurance athletics.

My research focused specifically on Ironman athletes because they are particularly prone to extreme exercise due to the duration of the event. Based on Collins' original format, an Ironman triathlon is composed of a 2.4-mile swim, a 112-mile bike, and a 26.2-mile run, undertaken sequentially and without interruption. This race takes competitors anywhere from seven to seventeen hours to complete, and training for an

Ironman takes a sizeable investment of time, energy, and expense. Rigid adherence to a training plan, as well as a nutrition plan, is imperative to complete an Ironman race. However, there is a distinction between dedicated and obsessive, and the current psychological tools available to assess exercise dependence may not be sensitive enough to distinguish between the two in the case of Ironman athletes. Nor are psychologists or coaches particularly attuned to the fine line that athletes toe day in and day out between health and addiction. One athlete's five-hour ride may be healthy for him/her, while another's fifty-minute run may be problematic; the line between healthy and unhealthy is determined by motivation and approach to training. And a mental health practitioner may not understand the rigid adherence to a training plan that is necessary to complete an Ironman, nor may a coach suspect an athlete's underlying compulsions to constantly compete. This work attempts to draw coaches, mental health practitioners, athletes, and loved ones into conversation with one another so endurance athletics can be celebrated for the healthy endeavors that they are—and not be used as a mask for an addiction, as they so often can become.

Endurance athletes are uniquely situated as potential exercise addicts due to their rigid and extensive training regime. This problem of potential addiction impacts the health and well-being of Ironman athletes and their families and should be of concern to their coaches and the psychologists who are treating, defining, and creating the screening tools for exercise addiction.

This basic question—where does a healthy hobby end and an addiction begin?—is the one I set out to answer and explain in *In Sickness and In Health*. In addition to formal interviews I conducted and questionnaires I administered in 2005–2006 with fifty-three athletes, I have spent the last five years intimately immersed in the triathlon subculture as both an athlete and a coach. I work for Carmichael Training Systems as a triathlon, cycling, and ultrarunning coach—an environment where both my co-workers and my clients are more than willing to share their experiences with the lure of exercise and the necessity of balance; in fact, this is a daily conversation between my co-workers and my athlete clients.

I am an authority on the subject of exercise addiction in endurance athletes because I'm an endurance athlete struggling with addiction; because I am a coach who counsels athletes daily, helping them cope with their addictions; and because I am an academic who has researched the topic of exercise addiction extensively. This tripartite approach uniquely situates me as a specialist on the subject of exercise addiction in endurance athletics.

This isn't just a book to watch the proverbial train wrecks, though. *In Sickness and In Health* will equip athletes, coaches, spouses, and friends with the tools necessary to evaluate the physiological progress of training and the psychological parameters to identify exercise addiction. Through interview data, psychological surveys, and suggestions for struggling athletes, this book offers the only personalized accounts of exercise addiction complemented with documented research findings. It is the first of its kind to not only address exercise addiction, which is so rampant among endurance athletes, but to also provide plans that optimally develop both the physiological *and* psychological conditioning of the athlete in order to reach the best possible performance. Athletes will be able to take control of their addiction and find proper coping skills which will enhance their life both inside and outside of the sporting realm.

The book is organized to introduce athletes, coaches, and interested readers to the topic of exercise addiction. In the first half, I present and explain the academic research concerning exercise addiction. In the second half, I equip athletes with tools they need to assess their own levels of addiction. The take-home piece of this book not only provides athletes with a book they can identify with, but also provides them with strategies, coping skills, and plans to optimize their future endeavors in the athletic world and beyond.

Chapter 1: Are We Crazy?

The pursuit of the slim, well-muscled body is not only an aesthetic matter, but also a moral imperative.... Fasting and self-inflicted physical punishment are the modern-day equivalents of medieval flagellantism. They are religious rituals, part of the immortality project of a secularized middle class that no longer believes in redemption of the soul and has turned instead to redemption of the body.

Murphy, 1990, p. 114

Are we crazy? Well, some would say yes; and I would tend to agree with them. Are we all crazy? Certainly not. The attitude with which we approach our training is crucial in determining this "crazy" factor. Do we turn to Ironman racing, ultrarunning, one more marathon, the next, the faster, the longer event, to "redeem" our body, as Murphy says? To give meaning and purpose to our life? To avoid confronting issues? There are a whole host of books out there about why we engage in physical activity: what we think about when we run, how to run faster, think less, think more, connect to the body, connect to the soul, give purpose to our life, etc.— but no book really nails endurance athletics down as a potentially unhealthy activity—and they don't because it's not **inherently**. Endurance athletics can **become** unhealthy, however—and it is a slippery slope and one that is easy and all too common to slide down. This book offers an account of how this slope has been constructed in our current cultural climate, some warning signs that danger may lie ahead for you, some tactics on how to avoid the potential pitfalls of exercise addiction, and tools for recovery.

As endurance athletes we face a paradox. Sane athletes can compete in seemingly insane events. The attitude with which an athlete approaches his/her training and not the amount of time an athlete spends training is the key component separating training from addiction. Throughout my research on exercise addiction in endurance athletes, I have found remarkably healthy attitudes and individuals who compete in 100-mile ultramarathons, and I have found very compulsive and rigid, and, yes, addicted athletes who race 5ks. The distance of the event does not dictate the extent to which athletes are "healthy" or "unhealthy." Instead it is the attitude with which they approach their training, and the motivation behind training and racing that determines their propensity for exercise dependence. While I have observed this as a coach and an athlete, I also have the statistics to substantiate this claim.

In my research for my Ph.D., I administered three psychological questionnaires to Ironman athletes and found that the higher an athlete scored on the question "I exercise to lose weight," the higher his/her overall exercise dependence score. Motivation factor number one becomes a warning sign for exercise addiction. I also found that athletes who were highly influenced by social attitudes towards appearance scored higher on exercise dependence scales (warning sign number two). While all of this is academic-speak, I intend to make my research accessible to athletes who have never taken a statistics class, while maintaining the academically rigorous nature of the research I have performed. In other words, this is a book not just about my experience as a coach, as an athlete, and as an observer of the wacky world of endurance athletics; it is also an academic account of this realm of athletics. And while it is academic, it is not just for academics. I seek to speak to athletes, coaches, and mental health practitioners alike, because if my work does not reach those it seeks to help, then I have not done justice to my project. I do not want to preach to the choir, nor do I want to talk to an empty room. It is my hope that someone reads his/her lived experience in these pages, that someone sees his/her potential addiction and how to solve it, that a loved one picks up these pages and learns how to help, or understands a little better the plight of his/her partner. Recognition is one goal of this book. If we can recognize ourselves in these pages, then we have a chance to change.

Do you or does someone you know, work with, or love suffer from chronic injuries, feel burned out, or have a hard time connecting with nontraining partners? Normalizing one's behavior by only spending time with other endurance athletes is a common trait of those suffering from addiction, because what we are doing doesn't seem crazy to anyone else already immersed in the activity. Thus perspective is a crucial component of determining the "crazy" factor or the extent to which someone may suffer from an exercise addiction. Just as those who frequent a bar regularly see nothing wrong with their community, ultrarunners, Ironman athletes, and endurance athletes of all ilk find camaraderie and companionship in their chosen endeavor. And while we don't tend to call what we are doing "crazy," others from the outside just might—jJust as if we were not immersed in the local bar scene at 11 a.m., we might label that behavior as not completely sane. We normalize our behaviors by surrounding ourselves with like-minded individuals. This is human nature. I am not claiming that this is a bad thing; I am merely offering athletes an opportunity to take one step outside of their "norm" to see what they are doing from an outsider perspective. Does this distance breathe new awareness into motivations and compulsions around training? Perhaps, perhaps not. Here's the good news, though: you may not be fully to blame. You are, after all, a product of your environment.

Cultural Context

An investigation of Ironman athletes not only examines the athletes themselves, but also the context in which their subjectivity is constituted. It is important to understand the current climate that gives rise to Ironman athletes, specifically in terms of gender, body ideals, and compulsions concerning weight, control, and addiction. Specifically, it is imperative to this study to account for the gendered, sexed, and fat-phobic context of the current U.S. climate and the simultaneous rise of the Ironman's popularity (four of the North America Ironman events sold out within twenty-four hours of the opening of registration, one year in advance of the race).

In the psychological literature, exercise addiction has been compared to eating disorders (Ogden, Veale, and Summers 1997; Yates, Leehey, and

Shisslak 1983) and compulsive addictions (Davis et al. 1995, Pasman and Thompson 1988). Adams and Kirby (1998), Anshel (1991), and Morris, Steinberg, Sykes, and Salmon (1990) documented the withdrawal effects associated with exercise cessation, including irritability and increased anxiety. Those who cannot stop working out, despite injury and illness, exercise to stave off the mood disturbances associated with taking time off. Currently the Diagnostic and Statistical Manual of Mental Disorders (American Psychiatric Association, *Diagnostic and Statistical Manual of Mental Disorders*, 1994) does not label compulsive exercise as its own illness or condition. However, the DSM-IV does define exercise as excessive (as a potential component of a primary eating disorder) "when it significantly interferes with important activities, when it occurs at inappropriate times or in inappropriate settings, or when the individual continues to exercise despite injury or other medical complications" (p. 546).

To date, studies conducted on excessive exercise have not examined elite athletes, but rather, runners (e.g., Slay, Hayaki, Napolitano, and Brownell 1998) and college students (Garman, Hayduk, Crider, and Hodel 2004). To date five social science studies have been published on specific populations of triathletes, but none was conducted on Ironman athletes exclusively. One study by Hilliard (1988) addressed the "triathlon scene," whereby Hilliard documented triathlon as its own unique subculture or *habitus*. Granskog (1992) looked at the way women were respected within the triathlon community. Bell and Howe (1988) examined mood profiles of triathletes, and Virnig and McLeod (1996) compared eating patterns of triathletes with eating patterns of distance runners. Triathletes demonstrated "healthier attitudes toward eating" (p. 82) in comparison to runners. Triathletes were happy (Bell and Howe) and healthy (Virnig and McLeod), or at least healthier than runners. The qualifier is important, particularly when considering the following study from the University of North Carolina.

DiGioacchino DeBate, Wethington, and Sargent (2002b) examined "body size dissatisfaction" and "subclinical eating disorders" in the population of triathletes. They differentiated their results by gender and found that approximately half of female triathletes and a third of male triathletes were preoccupied with food and bodily appearance. So while triathletes tested lower on an eating attitudes test (EAT), indicating a "healthier" outlook on food compared to distance runners (Vernig and McLeod 1996), they also were predominately preoccupied with food and body. They were only happy when they won, or at least placed well (Bell and Howe, 1988). These studies contributed to my understanding of the psychological profile of triathletes and informed my research questions, designed to probe further into the specific psychological constituency of exercise addiction among Ironman athletes. Exercise addiction does not exist in a vacuum; it is the product of a unique moment in time, specifically situated in the current U.S. context of fat phobia (Robinson, Bacon, and O'Reilly 1993) and rigid mandates for an appropriately gender body (Bordo 1993).

According to Scheper-Hughes and Lock (1987), "the individual body should be seen as the most immediate, the proximate terrain where social truths and social contradictions are played out, as well as a locus of personal and social resistance, creativity, and struggle" (p. 31). Ironmen embody these "social truths" commanding leanness and muscularity and social assumptions that posit fitness as the embodiment of health. But this story is not so simple as Ironmen emerging as the epitome of health or as the ultimate gender transgressor, in the form of female Ironmen. Ironmen present a much more complicated story, riddled with pathology, adherence to social expectations of gender, and the combination of the two in race results. This work examines Ironman athletes to understand the ways in which exercise addiction and gender performance create the corporeality of the Ironman athlete.

The significance of this study is to add research focusing on elite athletes, Ironmen specifically, to the literature on compulsive exercise, and to add the story of Ironman to the body of sport literature. I draw from contributions made in the field of postmodern gender theory to understand the culturally constructed bodies I examine in the Ironman racing realm. I look specifically at the ways in which gender norms affect

Ironman athletes and their motivation to train for and participate in the Ironman triathlon as a potential outlet for their exercise addiction.

To date, limited research focuses exclusively on triathlons, and none focuses specifically on Ironman. Triathlons vary in distance much like running events can span from 5 kilometers to a marathon (42 km). A sprint triathlon comprises a 400–800-meter swim, a 10–15-mile bike ride, and a 3–5-mile run. An Olympic-distance triathlon is a 1-mile swim, a 25-mile bike ride, and a 6.2-mile run. A Half Ironman is a 1.2-mile swim, a 56-mile bike ride, and a 13.1-mile run. An Ironman is a 2.4-mile swim, a 112-mile bike ride, and a 26.2 mile run. Thus Ironman is unique in that it differs from other triathlons due to its length. No research exists concerning exercise addiction in Ironman athletes, and, due to the length of the Ironman event, earlier investigations with triathletes may not capture the experience of Ironman competitors.

This study not only examines the culture of the Ironman, it also investigates the context of a sport which has been at the forefront of reinforcing gender norms by teaching about masculinity through force, power, and the observable absence of women (Messner and Sabo 1990). This historical legacy of the absence of women in sport must be acknowledged while describing the history and accounting for the climate of the Ironman triathlon—the site of this study. To responsibly report the influence of gender for the Ironman athlete, I drew from the rich scholarship of the gendering of sport, and I specifically employed a gendered perspective of sport theory.

Birrell and Theberge (1994) have been influential contributors to the rich scholarship mentioned above. They documented the ways in which gender norms have been both reinforced and challenged by athletes in the sporting realm. Women, Ironmen in particular, may, in fact, find personal empowerment through their physical and psychological struggles. However, such a simple assumption does not suffice for the complex inclusion and participation of women in sport. Indeed, Dworkin and Messner (1999), citing Bartkey, wrote,

By some standards, today's more muscular woman can be viewed as embodying agency, power, and independence in a way that exemplifies resistance to patriarchal ideals. However, just as within sport, women's bodily agency in fitness activities can be contradictory. Is this bodily agency resistant and/or empowering, or is the fit, muscled ideal simply the latest bodily requirement for women, a form of "self-surveillance and obedience" in service to patriarchal capitalism? (p. 351)

Bartkey challenged the notion that women earn empowerment by participating in sport simply due to the fact that sport has been historically a male domain. Transgressing this gender boundary is not necessarily progressive. Sometimes the transgression leads to further patriarchal "control" of the body—within or outside of the sporting realm. Agency is a central theme in this text. Agency in postmodern gender theory arises, according to Butler, in the "hiatus of iteration." When one ceases to act in accordance with the gender norm, that is agency. Women's participation in sport is a gender-transgressive behavior, but, according to Bartkey, is not necessarily agentic when one does so for the purposes of achieving a specific social aesthetic. Agency still remains in the discursive system that controls bodies and behaviors and not with the individual. This study investigates the extent to which the individual is affected by social ideals and are possibly "pathological" in their approach to exercise. I investigate the nature of Ironman athletes to understand the ways in which Ironman may very well be the "latest bodily requirement," or may in fact be "empowering," or a complex combination of the two.

Sport theorist Duncan (1994) unequivocally assessed the empowerment of women who "continually monitor their bodies for imperfections, who constantly diet, and/or who exercise to extremes," claiming that such women "are both physically and psychologically disempowered" (p. 54). According to Duncan's assertion then, are Ironman athletes (male and female) physically and psychologically disempowered? The answer to that question lies in the definition of "extreme." Is Ironman extreme? And who defines extreme? This study attempts to elicit a better understanding of whether or not Ironman athletes are empowered subjects or disempowered pseudoagentic beings in society—they still have agency, as they choose to race Ironman triathlons, but what are the influential factors informing this choice? Through an examination of both the definition of extreme (as defined by Ironman athletes themselves) and the motivating factors (why Ironman athletes choose to race), the results of this study answers the question: to what extent are Ironman athletes exercise addicts?

Female Ironmen interact with a gendered sport culture to write new truths about gender and endurance on their bodies. This investigation seeks to understand what those truths are and asks to what extent those messages are pathological. The Ironman athlete is a new athlete, and, potentially an ill athlete in an endurance sport that is popularly perceived as a healthy endeavor, even epitomizing health (according to ABC's *Wide World of Sports* televised coverage, 1980).

The social constructionist theory of gender informs my understanding of the ways in which gender is learned and enacted by both male and female Ironman informants. Using insights from Bordo (1989, 1993, 1997) and Grosz (1994), among others, I examine the extent to which social messages—discursively produced and perpetuated through the media—speak through the Ironman body. Specifically, I assess the extent to which Ironman athletes internalize social standards of beauty and the extent to which this internalization affects their level of exercise addiction.

Cultural theorist Bordo (1989) wrote, "The body [is] the locus of social praxis, as cultural text, as social construction, as the tablet on which new visions of an 'ecriture feminine' are inscribed" (p. 4). The body, the Ironman body, is not a discrete unit devoid of cultural commandments. Instead it is the very intersection of social mandates manifested in the physical body of Ironman athletes. This investigation seeks to understand what it is that Ironman athletes are saying with their bodies.

Cultural gender expectations manifest themselves on the body of each individual through the ritualized starving or the compulsive pumping of iron. Ironman athletes pride themselves on the fact that they can mold their bodies, their physiological energy systems, their body compositions, their psyches, into something that can sustain racing for hours on end.

Examining how Ironmen do and do not fit the description of compulsive exercisers, I situate the pathology of exercise addiction in the gendered context where the majority of individuals who suffer from anorexia are women (Mond, Hay, Rodgers, and Owen 2006; Yates et al. 1983), while men are being diagnosed with "bigorexia," a colloquial term to describe the obsessive gym-going male (Pope, Phillips, and Olivardia 2000). As such, this book presents a story of the Ironman athlete who exists in a particularly gendered realm of athletics as a culturally constructed subject internalizing a social aesthetic for thinness to the extent that an exercise pathology may be present.

Obligatory running, exercise addiction, and compulsive exercise all describe the phenomenon of individuals who are "addicted to exercise." As early as 1979, Sachs and Pargman published **Running Addiction,** in which they discussed both psychological and physiological addictions to running. Despite their description of withdrawal symptoms associated with cessation of activity, Sachs and Pargman still concluded that running is a healthy addiction and not a destructive one. According to them, running, as a positive addiction, encourages individuals to continue to work out and reap the benefits of aerobic exercise.

Since 1979, however, research on the topic of compulsive exercise contradicted Sachs and Pargman's findings. Bamber, Cockerill, and Carroll, in "The Pathological Status of Exercise Dependence" (2000), found that exercise addiction is actually detrimental to the health of affected individuals. Running can be a negative addiction when individuals run to stave off withdrawal symptoms when not engaged in physical activity. According to Sachs and Pargman (1979), a positive addiction is one that improves the health and well-being of the afflicted individual, whereas a negative addiction has detrimental affects on the addicted individual.

Biochemical explanations have been sought to explain the nature of the addiction to running. A variety of explanations for running addiction have been proposed, from endorphins to 5-Hydroxytryptamine levels accounting for the addictive nature of exercise as found in rats (Broocks, Schweiger, and Pirke 1991; Chaouloff 1989). The exact physiological explanation for compulsive exercise is beyond the scope of this book. However, the psychological classification of exercise addiction is essential to this project, as I use two validated psychological scales to measure exercise dependence and attitudes towards appearance in the gathering and analysis of my data: the Exercise Dependence Questionnaire (EDQ; Ogden, Veale, and Summers 1997) and Social Attitudes Toward Appearance Questionnaire (SATAQ-3R; Thompson, van den Berg, Roehrig, Guarda, and Heinberg 2004). Thus the history of the terminology, the definition, the diagnosis, and the understanding of exercise addiction in the field of psychology, as well as the iterations of the evaluation tools, are of paramount importance to this project.

In summary, this work takes a postmodern feminist approach (that bodies are discursively produced) to examine the Ironman athlete as a gendered subject in the masculine realm of sport and a current climate of thinness to assess the extent to which gendered notions of beauty affect athletes' propensity for participating in Ironman racing. The next chapter presents a story as to how it all began. It is a more in-depth literature review, and it is, perhaps, the most dense portion of this book. Once we wade through the work that has already been done in the field, I will present my own research findings, and then finally sum it up in the "take home" chapters of the text, applying and integrating the academic information to the lived experience of the endurance athlete.

Chapter 2: Timing is Everything: The Birth of Ironman, the Beginnings of Exercise Addiction

The three disciplines and associated theoretical constructs that inform my study of Ironman athletes derive from the history of women in sports, feminist theory, and psychology. Literature on the history of women in athletics is reviewed to contextualize the gendered climate of Ironman racing. Following this exploration into the world of sport, postmodern theorists Butler (1990, 1993, 1997), Bordo (1989, 1993, 1997), and Grosz (1994) are reviewed to understand both the bodies I examine and the systems that shape those bodies. Specifically, it is important to consider how these authors account for subjectivity in their postmodern theory to understand how Ironman bodies come into being as both individuals *and* cultural creations. Finally, the psychological literature concerning exercise addiction is reviewed to discuss the construct of "exercise addiction" as well as its responsible usage and appropriate application in describing the behavioral patterns exhibited by Ironman athletes.

Women in Sport: Historical and Theoretical Perspectives

The gendered climate of athletics sets a unique stage for gender norms, body constructs, and cultural expectations to manifest themselves in the athletes who participate in the Ironman triathlon. To fully understand the gendered climate of sport, the following is a brief history of women in sport, focusing on the exclusion and inclusion of women in the three disciplines that comprise the Ironman: swimming, biking, and running. Following this brief account of women in sport, the history of the Ironman race itself is reviewed to introduce the legacy of gender inclusion demonstrated by this race from its inception.

History of Women in Sport

While women have been historically "excluded" from sport, this is not a complete tale of the past. Spartan women could compete (Guttmann 1991), Victorian women engaged in regulated physical activity, albeit to offset the "burdens" of academic rigor (Vertinsky 1994a), and Bostonian women exercised to stave off illness (Vertinsky 1994a). Women played, they ran, they biked, they swam, they walked. Whether it was by covert means or by overtly asserting their presence in the sporting realm, they found ways of participating (Cahn 1994).

Despite not being "allowed" to run, women ran. They ran on their own and competed "illegally" by entering races under male pseudonyms (Kuscsik 1997). The history of women's participation in running events shaped the sentiments surrounding the acceptability of women's participation in later endurance events. Women pushed the boundaries of acceptability; they ran without numbers and refused to accept rejection when denied entry into race events. As such, women earned their rightful spot on the starting line, and the battle to get there both directly and indirectly shaped the acceptability of women in Ironman.

As early as 1896, a Greek woman by the name of Melpemone is said to have illegally run in the first Olympic marathon in Athens. She was not permitted to run due to her sex, but she ran anyway (Guttmann 1991). Not all female participation was prohibited, however. In the 1920s, women ran the 54-mile Comrades Marathon in South Africa and were hailed as heroes as much as the male winners (Kuscsik 1977). The history of women in sport is characterized by this ebb and flow of participation. At one moment women were accepted as competitors, and another moment staunchly denied access to the sporting realm.

The 1928 Olympic Games was the first moment when women were able to compete in the Summer Olympic Games' 800-meter event (Guttmann 1991). The half mile was the longest distance event open to women. However, the reporting of the event in newspapers across the country, including the *New York Times,* cast a long shadow over the acceptability of women in running events: "At the finish six of the runners were completely exhausted and fell headlong to the ground"; eleven women "collapsed" on the track, strewn about (as quoted in Guttmann). The fact that the female competitors were exhausted after their exertion was used against them, "proving" they were unfit for competition. This image of women exhausted and lying on the ground was unacceptable to the International Olympic Committee, already hesitant about including women in the Olympics. The sight of tired woman was unacceptable, while tired men were expected in sport, but issues of modesty and privacy precluded women from appearing exhausted after exertion (Cahn 1994). It was popularly believed and medically condoned that women who wasted energy on athletic competition necessarily diverted their vital energy from more gender-appropriate tasks such as birthing and caring for a family (Vertinsky 1994a). Consequently, women's track-and-field events were cut from the Olympic Games in 1932 (Guttmann). Thirty-two years later, by a narrow victory (26-22 International Olympic Committee vote; Guttmann, p. 203), the women's 800-meter event was once again allowed in the Olympic Games. It was not until 1982, however, that women could compete in the marathon event in the Olympic Games. The resistance to and ceaseless fight for participation in endurance sports for women pushed the boundaries of acceptability for female athletes. According to Guttmann, sport spectators (mostly male), entrenched in a rich history of the male preserve of sport, were uncomfortable with the image of exhausted women—it was perverse even, a sight likened to (pornographic) voyeurism. As Kuscsik (1977), an international runner herself, claimed, "When male runners collapsed en route in the marathon, it was called drama, but when women reached this physiological level, it was labeled 'frightful' " (p. 864). This double standard, this frightful sight, haunted female athletics for decades.

In the other sports involved in triathlon, namely the bike and the swim, women were also fighting for their right to participate. Guttmann (1991) and Shaulis (1996) comprehensively chronicled this fight. According to Guttman's research, as early as 1885 in France, women were invited to participate in swimming and bicycling events. In both sports, there was a "mixture of athleticism and femininity" (Guttmann, p. 102). Not only were women riding and swimming; in the nineteenth century women participated in long-distance pedestrian races. According to Shaulis, female walkers not only walked, their participation in sporting events challenged gender norms that women were not to display athleticism. Thus their mere presence in the athletic realm championed for women's rights (p. 5).

There was opposition to these early feminist pedestrians. In 1879 an outspoken male preacher commented on Madame Anderson's month-long walk, declaring that women should be celebrated for their strength as mothers and volunteers, not for their strength as walkers (as cited in Shaulis 1996). The preacher diplomatically did not deny the strength of women, but rather called for a shift of focus from the sporting (recreational realm) to the domestic.

The outspoken preacher was not alone. There has been much resistance to women's participation in sport. In the 1928 Olympic Games, Northwestern University swimmer Sybil Baur asked to swim against men in the Olympic backstroke. She was stoutly denied (Cahn 1994). Despite the strides being made by female athletes, the separate spheres of athletics were staunchly guarded. Women might compete, and might even be faster, but they were not to overtly beat men at their own game. This is what the coverage in the *Nation,* a newspaper covering women's swimming, conveyed to its audience (as cited in Cahn).

In 1868 British cycling tracks lost their licenses if women raced on their track (Guttmann 1991). However, France was more apt to allow women to partake in athletic events (Guttmann), demonstrated by the fact that women participated in cycling events. Perhaps the French influence in cycling had some effect on women's acceptance in Ironman racing, opening up the sport of cycling to women as an acceptable pastime. In France, England, and the United States, despite the fact that women were encouraged to partake in swimming and cycling activities, they were encouraged to limit their participation to recreation only, and sometimes that recreation was also limited (Hargreaves 1994).

According to sport historian Hargreaves (1994), "Cycling for women was described as an indolent and indecent practice which would even transport girls to prostitution; it was said to be an activity far beyond a girl's strength and one which made women incapable of bearing children" (p. 46). The link between cycling and prostitution is a stretch, but the threat alone was enough to keep women from riding. The promise of being barren was not worth the risk to most women. Hargreaves was not the only historian to document the threat of reproductive danger. Historian Mrozek (1987) also reported the belief that training women like men would lead them to be incapable of bearing children later in their life (p. 289). Thus the medicalization, the instilling of fear of the inability to reproduce, was enough to control women and keep them out of sport.

While many doctors cautioned against sport participation for women, female physician Lucy Hall disputed the medical model that cycling would be damaging to female reproductive organs. Lucy Hall was both a doctor and a cyclist, and in 1890 she deemed cycling beneficial for women. Indeed, she was not the only one to challenge the medical model (Lenskyj 1990). Roosevelt agreed with Hall and, in 1895, published a statement saying,

> There is no reason to think that a healthy woman can be injured provided she does not overexert herself by riding too long a time, or too fast, or up too steep hills, and provided she does not ride when common sense and physiology alike forbid any needless exertion, and provided also she does not get the bad habit of stooping over the handlebar. (Lenskyj 1990, p. 55)

With all of these caveats, there were many rationalizations to preclude women from riding. Not riding fast, not riding up hills, not riding too long, not "stooping" over the handlebars precludes women from both training and racing. Granted the permission to ride, they were to do so for pleasure and pastime only. Again, an ebb and flow of female participation characterizes the history of women in sport. At some moments they were able to participate, and at other times they were limited or excluded from sport.

Women who wanted to participate did so, despite the social norms that precluded them from competition. They would not be thwarted by their lack of opportunities to race in the Olympics and otherwise. They found alternate races in which to participate. In 1936 two women ran a 13-mile race up Pikes Peak in Colorado (Kuscsik 1977). And in 1959, twenty-nine-year-old Arlene Poerper ran up and down Pikes Peak. She was the first recorded woman to complete an organized marathon in the United States (Kuscsik).

Women demonstrated that they could participate without interfering with their ability to reproduce. According to sport historians Birke and Vines (1987), women were held back not by their biology, but rather by the social and cultural constraints placed upon their biology, and the proof of this is in the very fact that women are excelling in sport and doing so while remaining reproductive and healthy. Mrozek (1987) eloquently and succinctly captured this sentiment in his statement, "Woman's ability to perform effectively in defiance of the prevailing stereotypes should have been sufficient reason to question the stereotypes" (p. 292). The notion that women could not compete in sport was being challenged, and the tale of the Boston Marathon reflects this.

In 1966, Roberta Gibb Bingay requested an application to the Boston Marathon; she was denied (Kuscsik 1977). Race officials claimed that women could not run a marathon because they would injure themselves. She did not let that stop her, however. Crouching in the bushes, Bingay jumped out and ran without a number, finishing in 3:21, in the top third of the field. Having proven that she was able to run the distance without injury, she expected that the race director would then allow women to compete. He denied her participation in the race altogether, stating: "Roberta Gibb Bingay did not run *the* Boston Marathon; she merely covered the same route as the official race while it was in progress" (Kuscsik, p.

867). In 1967, Kathleen Switzer made it to the start line as a registered runner. She registered as K. Switzer and showed up in a baggy sweatshirt with her hair tied up and obscured by a hat. En route in the marathon, she was tackled and escorted off the race course by race officials enforcing the "no girls allowed" policy held by the Boston Athletics Association (Kuscsik). Finally, in 1971, the national chairman of the Amateur Athletic Union permitted "selected" women to participate in marathons. These "selected" women were, essentially, those who had already completed a marathon "illegally" (Kuscsik).

Seventy-six years after the founding of the Boston Marathon, in 1972, women were allowed to run—legally (Kuscsik 1977). However, the battle was not over. Women were required to provide medical certificates to be allowed to run a marathon, although men were not (Kuscsik, p. 870). Under the guise of protecting women and the propagation of the species, according to Kuscsik, male event directors took it upon themselves to monitor the health of their female athletes. Male race directors did not want to be liable for the collapse of female competitors; the same care (control) was not extended to male participants.

By the 1970s, the tide of women runners was becoming more visible. Rebellious predecessors set the stage for athletic acceptance among women. This acceptance came first as a separate but permitted standard set forth by the American Athletic Union (AAU). While the New York City Marathon, established in 1970, never had a policy against women racing, when the AAU sanctioned the race it stipulated that women could compete but had to begin ten minutes before the men in order to clarify that women were running their own race and not competing against the men (Kuscsik 1977). Without the power to challenge the Amateur Athletic Union rule, the New York Road Runners club was forced to abide by the rule. The female race participants were not. Having been granted the acceptance to race, women wanted more; they wanted to be considered athletic equals, and so they took their ten-minute lead by sitting down on the start line and waiting ten minutes for the "official" start of the race (Kuscsik). For the first time in racing history, women elected to take a ten-minute penalty for the sake of running with their competitors, both male and female (Kuscsik). The female competitors in 1970 challenged the power structure with their bodies, with their body language, and with their unanimous decision to compete *with* their male competitors. The message they conveyed was that they were competitors, too, and they set the stage for the female Ironmen to come.

The First Female Ironman

The arduous battle for athletic inclusion for women eased momentarily in 1979, when the first female competitor toed the starting line of the Ironman with thirteen male competitors, seemingly accepted as an equal. This history of women in sport, and endurance athletics in particular, culminates with the inclusion of women in Ironman. However, to fully understand the climate of Ironman as a specific sporting realm, one must first have a sound understanding of the history of the Ironman itself.

Fortuitously, Barry McDermott, a *Sports Illustrated* journalist, was in Oahu covering a golf tournament when he read about the Ironman Challenge in the local newspaper. He asked race director Collins if he could cover the event, at which point he was offered a spot in a support vehicle and spent fifteen hours documenting the event (Babbitt 2003).

McDermott (1979) observed the "addiction to inordinate amounts of exercise" each participant seemed to demonstrate, and he saw the Ironman as a "cult activity." He wrote, "That morning fifteen people, including a woman, had ignored the boundaries of sanity and started the contest," making note of the gender of one individual, Lynne Lemaire, the first female Ironman. Racing in third place, Dunbar, sporting a Superman outfit as he raced, was particularly concerned about Lemaire's positioning throughout the race. McDermott's report reads:

> When Lemaire [the only woman in the race] pedaled past Dunbar...[Dunbar] appeared startled, then asked a crew member, "Is she in the race?" Lemaire smugly turned and waved. She holds

the American women's cycling record for twenty-five miles. At five-foot-six and 148 pounds she is not a whole lot smaller than Warren, Dunbar, and Haller [race leaders], who are about five-foot-ten and 155 pounds. The woman cyclist closed to within five minutes. "Where's the girl?" Warren kept shouting. He started pumping harder.

Lemaire put up a good fight, raced her hardest and gave the other competitors good competition. She ended up placing fifth overall. McDermott characterized Lemaire as a courageous and talented athlete, not a female champion, not a pioneer, but an equal competitor. Other accounts of Ironman (Babbitt 2003) do not emphasize Lemaire's gender other than calling her the first female Ironman and a talented athlete. Her gender was not the selling point that earned her a place in Ironman history. Rather her performance trumped her gender, earning her recognition as a competitive equal in the Ironman competition.

While women competed despite their exclusion and medical management, the battle was hard fought and marked by moments of acceptance and rejection. By the 1970s, female participation was tolerated, albeit segregated, as typified by the New York Marathon. Ultimate acceptance came when women were seen as competitive equals. This acceptance, however, needs to be probed further lest acceptance be equated with empowerment or equality. Further examination reveals this issue to be more complex than female empowerment as actualized through sport participation.

This section has provided a brief historical overview of both the Ironman triathlon and the climate for female athletes prior to the inception of the Ironman. The gendered history of sport is a crucial component to this project because gender is a central construct in this project. The gender-*inclusive* nature of Ironman triathlon within the gender-*exclusive* nature of sport highlights the salient component gender plays in the identity of the athletes in this study.

Gender and the Body Inside and Outside of Sport

The research questions guiding this work focus on the Ironman athletes and the meaning and message of their purposefully constructed bodies. This review now considers the theoretical underpinnings that inform
the questions I ask and the ways in which I answer these questions and
interpret the data to examine *both* the bodies *and* the systems that shape
those bodies. Using a postmodern feminist approach to understanding
bodies as discursive entities, I look to the discourse in sport outlined by
sports-studies scholars, and outside of sport as articulated by feminist
scholars who theorize subjectivity and matters of the body, to understand
fully the bodies I am examining.

Heywood and Dworkin (2003) analyzed the position of the female
athlete as both an empowered being and as succumbing to the cult of
femininity. Analyzing media images and discourse surrounding the Wom-
en's National Basketball Association, the Women's United Soccer Association, and the fitness craze of the 1980s and 1990s, Heywood and Dworkin
situated the female athlete as straddling femininity and empowerment. In
some moments, she is strong, and, in others, she is a sexualized image on
the pages of a glossy magazine. In order to understand where female Ironman athletes fall along this spectrum, I first must examine the spectrum
itself.

Sporting women are not immune to the cultural mandates for thinness, and instead take their social mandates for perfection with them into
the sporting realm. Feminist theorist Duncan (1994) observed, "Women
who continually monitor their bodies for imperfections, who constantly
diet, and/or who exercise to extremes are both physically and psychologically disempowered" (p. 54). In this context it is important to look
at what motivates exercise. It is important to consider the purpose of the
exercise and whether the body is used as an object or whether the body is
used as an agent. If exercise is used to achieve a certain appearance—to
make the body look a certain way to others—then the body is an object. If
the exercise is used to make it possible for the body to do certain things—

then the body is an agent. If Ironman athletes use their bodies to achieve a certain body ideal, then they are using their bodies as objects; if they are using their bodies to complete races, then they are using their bodies as agents. Ironman athletes use their bodies to complete races. While all Ironman athletes use their bodies to complete races, the motivating factors that brought them to racing is important to unpack.

Similarly Bordo (1997) was skeptical of the female athlete as the necessarily empowered athlete. She wrote, "Women are exchanging their eating disorders for exercise compulsions, and their old addictions to controlling, masterful 'phallic' men for addictions to self-control and mastery of their own bodies" (Bordo 1997, p. 62). Exchanging eating disorders for exercise addictions is not a movement toward empowerment. Instead, it merely shifts the focus from eating to exercise. By addressing questions of the extent to which Ironman athletes demonstrate exercise addiction patterns and the extent to which they have internalized social norms for beauty may help to discern the extent to which Bordo's (1997) statement about exercise addiction as a substitute for eating disorders and self-mastery is applicable to Ironman athletes.

Bordo was cautious about lauding the hard work and diligence of a potentially destructive behavior (i.e., training for an Ironman). She believed that "food refusal, weight loss, commitment to exercise, and ability to tolerate bodily pain and exhaustion have become cultural metaphors for self-determination, will, and moral fortitude" (Bordo 1993, p. 68). Bordo was cautious about celebrating "strength" when this strength actually serves to disempower women and when empowerment is defined as the methodical monitoring, training, and sculpting of the body. These cultural metaphors are like misplaced modifiers; they praise behavior that is not praiseworthy, behavior that is actually self-destructive. Bordo's (1993) insight here is potentially applicable to Ironman athletes, who are presently celebrated as self-determined and strong individuals. Evaluating the extent to which they internalize cultural messages of beauty and their predilection to exercise addiction will illuminate the extent to which their food refusal, weight loss, and commitment to exercise is pathological.

Bordo (1989, 1993, 1997), Duncan (1994), and Heywood and Dworkin (2003) are not the only scholars evaluating the burgeoning number of female athletes and theorizing the meaning of their bodies in both sport and society. In 1993, Cole published her canonical article discussing the malleability of the body, specifically the ways in which women transform their bodies to conform to rigid mandates of femininity and beauty. The very fact that women *can* change their bodies in the attempt to mimic a social aesthetic (which changes over time and is different in different locales) simultaneously destabilizes the naturalized female body; the very body that has been cited as the cause of female subordination and also a potential path to liberation.

However, Cole (1993) recognized the prevalent role sport plays in this bodily morphology and simultaneously questioned its role in continuing to control the activities and the bodies of its female clientele. While Ironman athletes are not solely in the gym environment, the arguments that Cole (1993) makes about the motivations that drive women to the gym can be applied to Ironman athletes as well. It is possible that women (and men alike) flock to Ironman racing in the attempt to transform their body into a culturally valued and aesthetically pleasing body. Data gathered in interviews provides insight into the specific motivations of Ironman athletes and their opinions about beauty and their own bodies. To interpret these data, it is paramount to understanding the theories concerning bodies, beauty, female empowerment, and cultural conceptions of beauty that I outline here.

The bodies I interviewed, the bodies I theorized, are not static bodies. They are malleable. According to Moore (1997), "Built bodies are the ultimate expression of a postmodern belief in corporeal malleability" (p. 2). Through training, Ironman bodies are constantly shifting and morphing into something new, something more fit, less fit, faster, slower. The purpose of training, after all, is to shape the body. With this in mind, my work is attentive to both bodies *and* the systems that shape and reshape our bodies. For this reason I rely heavily on postmodern and postcolonial feminist theory to understand the Ironman athlete and the systems that influence and actualize Ironman athletes.

Reviewing influential postmodern theorists is important to delineate the historical framework that now shapes the conception of the body in contemporary feminist inquiry. According to Flax (1990), embodiment comprises how we feel, what we think, and what the world tells us: "it is simultaneously somatic, psychic, and discursive" (p. 98). Flax's tripartite theory covers a wide range of influential factors concerning embodiment. What it offers in breadth, it lacks in depth. It is, however, an apt place to begin the discussion of embodiment, as it exposes the multiple ways in which embodiment occurs. Insights from Butler (1990, 1993, 1997), Grosz (1994), and Bordo (1989, 1993, 1997) complement and expand upon Flax's theory. Each theorist posits something different as to how social influence operates on the body to create its materiality, thus expanding upon Flax's notions of embodiment. Butler (1990, 1993, 1997) cited a rigid system of punishment that reinforces a narrow range of appropriate gender behaviors. Grosz (1994), in contrast, posited that discourse operates strictly on the surface of the body. Bordo (1989, 1993, 1997) believed that the body is targeted directly and influenced deeply by social discourse. I weave in other influential thinkers, but I take these three theorists to be representative of the philosophical and sociological theories influential in and representative of postmodern feminist theory and the ways in which embodiment and subjectivity are conceptualized in the field. In this study I came to understand my subjects and their experiences as gendered Ironman athletes through the lens offered by postmodern feminist theory.

The Historicity of the Body in Feminist Discourse

Discussion of the postmodern body emerges from an earlier context of structuralist feminist theory. Spelman (1988) summarized conceptions of the body in structuralist feminist theory by critiquing the negative association articulated by Friedan's (1964), de Beauvoir's (1949/1989), and

Firestone's (1970) connection between the body and oppression. Carrying the argument one step further, Spelman reasoned that if the body is the root of oppression, shedding the body becomes the path to liberation.

A structuralist account of identity posits that a biological body (male/female) creates a given identity in the mind, which then is reified in the body. "Primary" sex characteristics shape constructs in the brain (as delineated by Gilligan, for example, in *In a Different Voice,* 1993). Mental conception of identity further reifies the body construct from which the persona (female) was originally perceived as being crafted (as being born a girl). Structuralist feminists challenge the necessary link between biological sex and social gender. They posited that biological sex is based on a mutually exclusive binary system of sex wherein every individual is either male or female and determined such at birth. Gender is defined as behaviors often associated with male and female descriptors. In challenging the behaviors but neglecting to critically examine biological sex, structuralist feminists inadvertently reified the body as a prediscursive entity. Postmodern feminists, following Butler, recognized this gross oversight that the body can never exist outside of discourse and sought to theorize about the body prediscursively. They concluded that there is no prediscursive body nor a "pure" entity or truth of the body.[1] All bodies are shaped by social interaction. Postmodern feminists challenged the central tenet upon which structuralist feminists waged their argument. This is how the body entered into the realm of social construction.

Accounting for the Gendered Body, the Female Ironman

The body comes into being through interaction, through socialization, and through powerful hegemonic systems. Sport scholar Pamela Moore (1997) wrote, "malleable flesh [is] abstractly molded by power" (p. 5). This literature review examines the systems of power that shape the

---

1. *This premise, however, is not accepted in the discipline of psychology a la Gilligan. Thus there is a point of discord in the different disciplines I integrate in my work. This does not, however, detract from the contributions made by each discipline to this project.*

bodies of both male and female Ironman athletes to fully understand the meaning and motivation of the Ironman body.

This body is a carefully constructed body; it is not prediscursive, nor is it isolated as an Ironman body. It is created in training, in interacting, inside and outside of the Ironman racing realm. Each interaction influences the bodies of the Ironman athletes under investigation, and, therefore, the interactions of the participants with the interviewer are also part of that construction. Thus, this project does not present a singular truth about Ironman athletes; instead, it presents an amalgamation of stories, statistics, and interpretations concerning the experience of Ironman athletes and the cultural climate that celebrates Ironman accomplishments. Donna Haraway (1991) affirmed "bodies are not born; they are made… their boundaries materialize in social interactions" (p. 208). These social interactions shape who Ironman athletes are, and one component of that subjectivity is their gender.

Interactions generate gender. According to Kessler and McKenna (1978/1985), "secondary gender characteristics and genitals are important cues, but they are never sufficient for making a gender attribution. Whether someone is a man or a woman is determined in the course of interacting" (p. 17). According to Butler, "there is no reference to a pure body which is not at the same time a further formation of that body" (1993, p. 10). Meaning is generated through the very description of that which is attempting to be described. In summary, the body becomes the mode of production, the vehicle through which description is articulated and enacted. Bodies are shaped by descriptions, and discourse defines and regulates behaviors.

Gender is discursively produced.[2] Norms shape bodies, shape conceptions of bodies, and thus shape "appropriate" gender identifications.

2. French theorist Foucault (1980) offered a helpful definition of discourse that historically situated the arguments in postmodern feminist theory. Foucault also offered a comprehensive account of what precisely influences the body in discourse. Foucault defined the "social" upon which other postmodern feminists build their theory of corporeality. His insights have shaped the formation of postmodern thinking, particularly in terms of corporeal construction. Foucault cited discourse as constituting corporeality. Discourse is a practice that forms the object of which it speaks. Discourse operates on a systemic

These identifications are predicated on a coherent sex and gender binary, whereby gender forms from a supposed substantive sex. Bodies are formed through the sexing/gendering practices of social order instantiated at birth and perpetuated throughout life. While this study uses the terms "male" and "female" to communicate the experience of Ironman athletes, it does so with a critical perspective of the social construction of the sex/gender system. Enacting gender simultaneously shapes bodies—Ironman bodies not excluded. As Butler (1990) articulated, sex and gender are mutually constitutive of one another. And social institutions affect the conception of appropriate feminine attributes. Social institutions mark bodies, judge bodies, and inform identities.

Postmodern theorist Butler (1990, 1993, 1997) offered insight into the ways in which the mind and body are both shaped by social interaction and mutually influence one another. Butler's theories (1990, 1993, 1997) are predicated on Foucaultian (1980) contributions. Butler has written the canonical texts of postmodernity in feminism in which she claimed that each person nominally acts out his/her gender as deemed appropriate by social standards in relation to a gendered ideal. Systemic adherence to this rule creates the illusion of gender as a stable entity of being, often informed and dictated by sex located in the genitalia. Sex does not determine gender, but rather gender and sex are both socially constructed. By repeatedly responding to the word "girl," a person learns to enact all that "girl" entails; in so doing the exteriority of femininity reifies the belief of a core female interiority. Gender is conceived, created, and perpetuated by actors in the social realm. Gender is not a "natural" process that necessarily develops from "sex" (Butler 1990). Butler challenged the ontological root of gender. She stated,

---

level whereby, according to the French philosopher, power acts by laying down the rule: power's hold on sex is maintained through language, or rather through the act of discourse that creates, from the very fact that it is articulated, a rule of law. It speaks, and that is the rule. (83) Discourse shapes bodies by creating their very subjectivity. According to Foucault, by identifying discourse, a polemic of power may be introduced to establish a resistance to discursive methods.

Gender is the repeated stylization of the body, a set of repeated acts within a highly rigid regulatory frame that congeal over time to produce the appearance of substance, of a natural sort of being. A political genealogy of gender ontologies, if it is successful will deconstruct the substantive appearance of gender into its constitutive acts and locate and account for those acts within the compulsory frames set by the various forces that police the social appearance of gender (p. 33).

By challenging the supposed "natural" root of gender, Butler destabilized the predetermining factor for gender: sex. Identifying this performative practice reveals that there is, in fact, no history to gender apart from its social construction. Sex is as much of a social construction as is gender; sex is already gendered. A body is labeled female: thus an individual learns to act female through a system of punishment and reward (Butler 1990). Throughout the course of this learning process an individual comes to identify as female. This procedure occurs systemically by the compliance of individuals who perpetuate the gender order. The regulated exteriority of gender shapes the "interiority" of sex, simultaneously gendering, sexing, and sorting bodies.

Critics of postmodern theorists ask: if bodies are constructed, sexed, gendered, policed, and always already culturally embedded, how then is agency accounted for, or is it? Butler countered, "Agency is the hiatus in iteration" (1997, p. 87). Agency is asserted when one removes oneself from the compulsive repetition of gendered acts through conscious action. Is the link between the mind and the body so fluid, as Butler would assert, that any mental "hiatus in iterability" alters body morphology? Understanding bodies as constructed enables a reconstruction of physicality. However, one cannot always recreate their materiality, their body. Skin pigmentation, disabled bodies, and XY-chromosome-carrying individuals cannot transform into different skin colors, able-bodied individuals, or fetus-carrying men by thinking it so. However, Butler enabled a view of a hierarchically organized sorting schema as socially constructed. But

an understanding of performativity does not change the physical conse-
quences, particularly of disability and pregnancy.

Bodies that experience specific treatment based on embodiment
would dispute the pure social construction of their physicality. Disabled
persons are constrained by certain biological and physiological circumstances. Although social order has stigmatized disability and has restricted
mobility for wheelchair-bound individuals, there is still a materiality
within which the disabled body is working. Butler did not adequately address this in her theory of performativity.[3] She allocated too much agency
to the mind and social interaction in the creation of the text of the body.
Even so, Butler's theories of performativity still offer a valuable and comprehensive account of sex and gender and the ways in which Ironman
athletes have been influenced and affected as gendered subjects. Thus,
moving beyond the discussion of the postmodern feminist account of gender, it is also important to review the theories that account for a cultural
aesthetic of thin beauty to further develop the theoretical understanding
of the systems that shape the bodies I examine.

Butler (1990) offered a way to conceptualize Ironman athletes as
agentic creatures, existing in their mind and body, and challenging and, at
times, conforming to social expectations of gender. At all times, though,
through training and racing, Ironman athletes shape their bodies purposefully and simultaneously shape their identities—as interview data will
show in the next chapter.

Ironman bodies tell a story. They are socially constructed bodies, as,
according to Butler, there is no essential characteristic to any being; "there
is no body prior to its marking" (1993, p. 98). The materiality of the body
is always socially constructed, and the Ironman body is no exception; it
too is socially constructed and imbued with cultural meaning and cultural
capital. The aim of this study is to decipher the meaning and to clarify the
message.

---

3. *Other theorists have critiqued both Butler (1990, 1993, 1997) and Haraway (1991)
for their inattention to disability as a corporeal reality apart from performativity and
situated knowledge. See Samuels, 2002; Nast and Pile, 1998; and Kirby, 1996.*

Philosopher Grosz (1994) loaned insight into what Ironman bodies could be saying with their corporeality through her explanation of how bodies come into being. Grosz wrote, "Social inscriptions on the surface of the body generate a psychical interiority—[a] movement from the outside in" (p. 115). The social inscription of the Ironman athlete, the way in which this athlete is received by his/her family, his/her competitors, his/her training partners, shapes his/her very understanding of himself/herself. Thus, Grosz's theory of embodiment proposed a fixed and fluid subject, as social inscriptions are malleable and temporally and spatially dependent. Ironman athletes receive different messages about their bodies at different moments in time and different locales. On the starting line, for example, if a competitor remarks, "Wow, you look fast," that may be message enough to spark a good race by instilling a belief in one's speed. The converse, however, is also possible.

Grosz (1994) offered a time-conscious account of corporeality. In *Volatile Bodies,* Grosz theorized about the body in psychoanalytic terms. A postmodern theorist informed by Freud (1930), Foucault (1980), Butler (1990, 1993, 1997), Irigaray (1985), and Cixous (1976), Grosz outlined her own assertions about the place of the body in feminist theory and situated the body in a larger social sphere. Grosz (1994) made explicit the interaction between body and culture. She stated, "The body is not opposed to culture, a resistant throwback to a natural past; it is itself a cultural, *the* cultural, product" (p. 23). Grosz defined the body as a "sociocultural artifact" (p. 115). As articulated earlier, other feminist scholars reiterated the historicity of the body in similar ways, popularizing the view of the body as socially and temporally constructed. Ironman athletes are no exception here as they purposefully create their body over time and through training.

In accordance with Butler (1990, 1993, 1997), Grosz (1994) asserted that sex is already gendered; bodies are always inscribed with socially constructed meanings. She cautioned feminists who rally around gender about reifying the genesis of a singular biological "woman" and mitigating the potential for individuality. Grosz situated subjectivity in the very malleability of the body itself, on its socially constructed surface, not in the reification of a socially constructed identity. What this means for Ironman athletes is that their ability to change, to be fit or unfit, as the case may be, is at the heart of their subjectivity as an Ironman athlete.

Beyond Butler: Cultural Aesthetic

To further understand the specifics of the cultural construction of the gendered body, it is important to critically examine the insights of Knapp (2003), Riley (1988), and Bordo (1989, 1993, 1997), who studied the specific cultural aesthetic that leads, in some cases, to the anorexic and to the exercise addict. According to Knapp, the body is the materiality upon which cultural meaning is inscribed.

Culture is written on the body, in this view, encoded on it. Fat, thin, sculpted, adorned, starved, stuffed, the female body is a kind of text which, properly deconstructed, may tell us a lot about how women are seen in the culture, and what they grapple with. (p. 100)

Culture can literally shape the materiality of body, as in the case of anorexic women and women who undergo cosmetic surgery. The internalization of cultural mandates of a prescribed beauty physically alters the materiality of the body, whether through food or makeup or plastic surgery. Culture acts on the mind as well as on the body in the case of anorexics who, through willful starvation, carve out the materiality of their body.

Cultural theorist Bordo (1989, 1993, 1997) also situated the body in social discourse. Bordo defined the body as "the locus of social praxis, as cultural text, as social construction, as the tablet on which new visions of an 'ecriture feminine' are inscribed" (Bordo 1989, p. 4). Bordo believed that the body is a malleable entity formed by discourse, which set the groundwork for her subsequent claims: "we learn the rules directly through bodily discourse: through images that tell us what clothes, body shape, facial expression, movements, and behavior are required" (Bordo 1993, p. 170). In contrast to Butler (1990), who asserted that the body is shaped through a system of repeated punishments and rewards, Bordo believed that the body is shaped through social discourse directly. Bordo's theories are distinct as she theorized at the surface of the body and its interiority rather than at the level of mind, as Butler (1993) does. Butler claimed performativity reifies identity constructs. Bordo (1993), instead, cited discourse and hegemony acting on the body, perpetuated through media images of idealized women as the nemesis of female liberation.

As such, Bordo's (1989, 1993, 1997) resolution to patriarchal oppression is hypothesized at the site of the body, since the body was cited as the original cause of subordination. According to Butler (1997), it is also the site for liberation, so long as women are unwavering in their diligence to resist gender oppression through their body, through the choices they make ,and through their purposeful creation of their morphology. This work includes the skepticism of fitness as libratory when it is in the service of a cultural aesthetic that serves to disempower women. Thus Bordo (1993) offered a model to conceptualize the gendered body of the Ironman athlete as a female body that challenges a male norm in sport, and as a female body that works tirelessly to become the most lean and powerful athletic machine it can be. However, the question remains: is this work for the purpose of obtaining a cultural aesthetic, or is it a route to liberation and equal treatment for the women who have for decades been excluded from sport?

Ironman bodies are not only a unique entity but are also a representation of the systems that shapes their bodies. Through resistance to iteration, according to Butler (1997), or nonconformity, according to Bordo (1993), individuality may be asserted. This individuality, this Ironman identity, is not a fixed and immutable attribute, however.

Bodies are constantly moving through this world, interacting, influencing, and being influenced by interactions. As our bodies collide spiritually, emotionally, intellectually, physically, and sexually with other bodies, our sense of self is influenced, challenged, and modified. Identities cannot be captured in static qualifiers. Descriptors often imply the immutability of identity as arrested in a specific moment in time. In actuality, we are always changing, affected by time and influenced by our social interactions. Our corporeality influences our identity, and every embodied interaction impacts our cognitive sense of self. This is not to imply a distinct severance of mind from body, but rather to suggest that our bodily experiences affect our comprehension of our self, our identity. Thus the Ironman bodies presented are situated in a particular moment in time and are not to be interpreted as a singular truth representative of all Ironman athletes.

The purpose of this review of postmodern gender theory is to comprehend the conversation that has existed in feminist theory concerning the construction of gender. While postmodern theories have helped feminists conceptualize the body without further reifying it as the mode of oppression for women, there remain limitations to postmodern theory. Postmodern theorists posit that a socialized identity constructs sexed bodies at birth; this descriptor (male/female) shapes the materiality of the body, which in turn creates identity in the mind, reifying a bodily truth. Postmodern theorist Butler (1990, 1993, 1997) claimed that through performativity, the process can be reversed. Psychosomatic illnesses, for example, demonstrate how powerful the mind can be in creating physical symptomology. Any athlete knows that optimal performance, referred to as "the zone," is only achieved when the mind is quieted. The chasm between the mind and body is neither as deep nor as wide as postmodern theorists have claimed it to be. Postmodernists have asserted that there is no gap, there is only mind, that the body is discursively constructed with no prediscursive reality. Conceptualizing the body as text with the mind as the actor is merely circular and dualistic; it does not help us conceptualize the experiential truth of a mind-body synchronism.

The psychological literature contributes to our understanding of the mind of the triathlete, the exercise addict, the anorectic, and complements the synchronicity between mind and body that postmodernist theory falls short of presenting. As the previous pages have delineated, the mind can never be separated from the body. No mind exists without a body, and no place is this more evident than in the pathological exercise addict presented in the psychological literature.

The Psychology of Exercise Dependence

This project uses a postmodern feminist approach to understand the bodies of Ironman triathletes. These bodies are discursively produced, and insights offered by sports scholars are needed to contextualize the gendered climate in the sporting domain, as well as the insights of feminist scholars who identify and articulate the pressures endured by women in this weight-conscious culture. The sports literature and feminist literature conjoin in the following discussion of the psychological disorder called exercise dependence. In the field of psychology the dialogue concerning *exercise dependence* is relatively new (first used in 1970), and exercise dependence remains a somewhat contested construct. The term "exercise addiction" originated outside of psychology and only recently has begun to find its way into the psychological literature. As excessive exercise patterns were investigated, research shifted away from descriptive accounts of exercise addiction and towards the quantitative investigations of exercise dependence.

Hausenblas and Symons Downs (2002a) published a comprehensive literature review of work in the field of psychology concerning exercise dependence from 1970 to 1999. They documented seventy-seven articles addressing exercise dependence and eleven articles discussing exercise withdrawal. They separated their results into three categories: studies that compared exercise-dependent individuals to eating-disorder patients, studies that compared exercise-dependent individuals to "normal" exercisers, and studies that compared exercisers to nonexercisers. They found no consensus of opinion concerning exercise dependence, diagnoses, or criteria.

While many studies contributed invaluable information to the burgeoning field of exercise dependence, none distinguished exercise from training nor focused solely on professional or elite athletes. The following literature review is organized chronologically as well as topically, beginning with early descriptions of the phenomenon of exercise addiction and moving to the diagnosis and creation of diagnostic tools. Then come studies that challenge the psychological significance of exercise addiction—calling it a positive addiction and negating the need for diagnosis and treatment. Thus exercise addiction presents an intriguing debate in the field of psychology, one in which this study is firmly entrenched.

As this is a multidisciplinary study, it is important to define terminology used in each discipline. Presently the DSM-IV uses *dependence* and *abuse of substances* rather than *addiction* to determine psychological pathology in individuals. "Addiction" is considered a behavioral term and not a diagnostic term. Addiction is the state of being physically dependent upon a drug and, in general, addiction implies increased tolerance to a drug and physical and psychological dependence so that withdrawal symptoms occur when administration of the drug is stopped (DSM-IV-TR). In the following discussion, it is important to understand that "dependence" is a diagnosis, whereas "addiction" is still considered a description of a behavioral pattern in the field of psychology. The following criteria are used to make a diagnosis for dependence according to the DSM-IV-TR:

A maladaptive pattern of substance use, leading to clinically significant impairment or distress, as manifested by three (or more) of the following, occurring at any time in the same twelve-month period:

1. Tolerance, as defined by either of the following:
   a. A need for markedly increased amounts of substance to achieve intoxication or the desired effect
   b. Markedly diminished effect with continued use of the same amount of the substance
2. Withdrawal, as manifested by either of the following:
   a. The characteristic withdrawal syndrome for the substance (refer to criteria A and B of the criteria sets for withdrawal from the specific substances)
   b. The same (or a closely related) substance is taken to relieve or avoid withdrawal symptoms
3. The substance is often taken in larger amounts or over a longer period than was intended

4. There is a persistent desire or unsuccessful efforts to cut down or control substance use
5. A great deal of time is spent in activities necessary to obtain the substance (e.g., visiting multiple doctors or driving long distances), use the substance (e.g., chain-smoking), or recover from its effects
6. Important social, occupational, or recreational activities are given up or reduced because of substance use
7. The substance use is continued despite knowledge of having persistent or recurrent physical or psychological problems that is are likely to have been caused or exacerbated by the substance (e.g., current cocaine use despite recognition of cocaine-induced depression, or continued drinking despite recognition that an ulcer was made worse by alcohol consumption (p. 197).

In this study the substance used is exercise. Psychologists use this definition of dependence to investigate whether or not exercise can be a behavior one can depend on in an unhealthy way. The debate in the field of psychology is central to this study, because to investigate and apply a construct, it is important to understand how the construct came into being. Just as unpacking gender is central to the gendered critique in this study, delineating the history of exercise dependence in the field of psychology is of paramount importance to its use and application with the particular subset of Ironman athletes under investigation.

Early Signs of Dependence

Orthopedists, not psychologists, were the first to document the phenomenon of exercise addiction. Repeatedly, they witnessed the deleterious effects of exercising in excess because those suffering from exercise addiction were unable to cease exercising until severe bodily injury hampered their routine. At this point, injured runners (exercise addicts) sought treatment in order to return to exercise as fast as possible. In 1979, Morgan, a professor of physical education and member of American College of Sports Medicine, documented this phenomenon. In this early observation about exercise addiction, Morgan likened the exercise addict to the drug addict. "The runner who appears in the physician's office on crutches or in a wheelchair as a result of the crippling effects of excessive running can be compared to the hard-core drug addict who overdoses" (p. 58). Citing Freud's (1930) "pleasure principle" as a possible explanation for the addiction, Morgan described how running 1 mile produces a positive emotional state, and the runner who craves more and longer feelings of pleasure extends his/her run to 2, 3, and 4 miles, compounding the effects of the pleasurable stimuli while simultaneously displaying early signs of addictive behavior.

Morgan (1979) based his "diagnosis" of exercise "addiction" on mileage and the Freudian pleasure principle. He claimed that runners who ran 70–100 miles weekly were "probably" addicted to exercise. However, he offered a caveat allowing for the aberration of 30–50-mile-per-week runners who were addicted and the few 100-miler runners who were not. Morgan does not explain why this phenomenon occurs other than "losing perspective," nor does he offer any explanation as to what enables a 100-mile-a-week runner to not become addicted. While Morgan began the discussion of exercise addiction, albeit from the perspective of a professor of physical education and not from a background in psychology, he left many questions concerning exercise addiction unanswered, including why one becomes addicted and what qualifies as addiction.

Drawing from Morgan's insight of the addictive nature of exercise, Sachs and Pargman (1979), also from a physical-education department, investigated further into what happens to exercise addicts who cease exercising. By interviewing twelve adult males who varied in their commitment to running, Sachs and Pargman (1979) identified both psychological and physiological symptoms of withdrawal from exercise, including bloatedness, uneasiness, irritability, tension, and guilt. In addition to the inability to rest or their compulsion to train through injury, exercise addicts displayed noticeable withdrawal symptoms when they were unable to work out. Sachs and Pargman (1979) defined the running addict again in terms of time and distance; for them, exercising six to seven days per week for an hour or more was one component of their tripartite diagnostic criteria. The other two criteria included exercise as an "integral" part of one's existence and intense withdrawal symptoms when a workout was missed. Sachs and Pargman (1979) offered the earliest diagnostic criteria for exercise addiction based on their in-depth interviews and identified the criteria as (1) time commitment, (2) withdrawal, and (3) the centrality of the activity, three of the seven diagnostic criteria for dependence, according to the DSM.

Anshel (1991) examined the "psychological characteristics and behavioral tendencies" of exercise addicts. While Anshel's article was originally published in the *Journal of Sports Behavior* and not a psychological journal, it is one of the first quantitative accounts of exercise addiction. He operationally defined exercise addicts as those who spent more than fifteen hours per week exercising continuously over a twenty-week period. Using this criteria and a Likert-scale questionnaire, Anshel conducted an analysis of variance (ANOVA) to compare exercise addicts to male and female nonaddicts and found that exercise addiction was a unique symptomology and displayed distinguishable characteristics. Anshel found addicted exercisers were significantly different from their nonaddicted counterparts in the following four ways: exercise addicts were more stressed prior to exercise, experienced a high level of mood elevation following exercise, were more "depressed, anxious, and angry" when a workout session was missed, and exercised despite injury or illness.

Anshel (1991) also was able to isolate gender variables, deducing that "male addicts revealed markedly higher levels of happiness and competence while feeling less mentally stressed than addicted females and both male and female nonaddicts" (p. 3). In other words, males displayed more exercise-dependent characteristics than females.

Anshel (1991) imposed an operationally defined criteria for exercise addiction to examine behavioral and psychological differences in exercise addiction, namely the amount of time spent training; however, when time alone is the single marker of exercise addiction, committed athletes, Iron-man athletes, and high-caliber athletes may be falsely pathologized.

In an exploratory study of withdrawal amongst competitive athletes, Crossman (1987) studied 31 competitive runners and 20 competitive swimmers. Crossman administered Polivy's Mood Scale and Spielberger, Gorsuch, and Lushene's (1970) State Anxiety Scale before a training session, after a training session, and on the second and fifth day of training cessation. Crossman found that males and higher-caliber athletes had more mood disturbances during exercise cessation than females and athletes at a lower level of competition, reporting similar results as Anshel's (1991) findings that males demonstrate higher exercise dependence patterns. While Crossman included competitive athletes in his study, he did not report the specific level of mood disturbance for high caliber female athletes or low-level male athletes.

The lack of research on this topic using competitive athletes may be due to the fact that examining exercise cessation among athletes is difficult. Morris et al. (1990) found it challenging to draw subjects to a study of temporary withdrawal from running, as most committed runners would not voluntarily cease exercise. Morris et al. recruited subjects in a newsletter posting the results of the 1986 St. Albans Marathon. Male subjects were selected if they ran at least three times per week and a minimum of 10 miles per week for three months and were willing to participate in the study for a six-week period. The forty male subjects were separated into two groups: a "deprived" group and a "control" group. The deprived group agreed to not run for two weeks and not to substitute any other activity for running. The control group continued with their typical running regime. Subjects completed the twenty-eight-item General Health Questionnaire as well as the six-item Zung anxiety and depression scales weekly. Through ANOVA and analysis of covariance (ANCOVA), researchers were able to demonstrate that withdrawal symptoms including irritability, anxiety, and decreased mood state accompanied exercise cessation.

Case Study

Griffiths (1997) documented the case of a twenty-five-year-old female who prioritized running over all other obligations in life, including work and family. When she began running, she covered shorter distances, and over time she extended her runs to feel the same levels of satisfaction postworkout. She had to run 8 miles to feel like she had after running 3 miles months earlier. While the training effect accounted for some of this "tolerance," the increased amount of stimuli to obtain the same level of satisfaction, the training effect did not account for all of it. By "training effect," I mean that her cardiovascular system and aerobic energy system became more efficient over time, and she no longer grew as tired running 3 miles when she began her daily running regime. As such, the training effect accounts for her cardiovascular adaptation to the exercise, but not her psychological "tolerance." Griffiths presented this case to dispel prior research lauding exercise addiction as a healthy addiction, a positive addiction. Instead Griffiths presented a tragic tale, in his opinion, of a distinctly negative addiction, one marked by the loss of friends, financial debt, and dissolving a relationship with a significant other.

Developing Diagnostic Criteria and
Measuring Exercise Dependence

Following the documentation of the phenomenon of exercise dependence, be it from sports-studies scholars, physicians, or psychologists, psychologists sought to quantify the symptoms of exercise dependence through the use of psychological questionnaires. Chapman and DeCastro (1990) developed the "running addiction scale," validated on forty-seven subjects and focused on the singular activity of running. The Obligatory Exercise Questionnaire (Pasman and Thompson 1988) evaluated all forms of exercise, including, but not limited to, aerobics, running, cycling, swimming, and weight lifting, and was a substantial start to the development of the instrumentation used to evaluate exercise dependence.

Following the development and validation of the Obligatory Exercise Questionnaire, Ogden et al. (1997) developed the Exercise Dependence Questionnaire (EDQ), one of the biggest advances in measuring and diagnosing exercise dependence. Ogden et al.'s questionnaire consists of a total score and eight subscales answered on a five-point Likert scale, with one indicating strong disagreement and five strong agreement. The eight subscales include: interference with social/family/work life; positive reward; withdrawal symptoms; exercise for weight control; insight into problem; exercise for social reasons; exercise for health reasons; and stereotyped behavior.

Ogden et al. (1997) developed and validated the EDQ using two sets of subjects. The first set used 131 self-described exercise addicts who were involved in the development of the original eighty-six items. The second set of 449 individuals reported exercising more than four hours per week and were involved in the validation of the final questionnaire. The first set of subjects completed unstructured questions about their feelings and cognitions concerning their exercise behavior. The original eighty-six items were the result of themed analysis of responses to broad questions. The second set of subjects completed the resulting eighty-six-item questionnaire. Factor analysis produced nine factors and resulted in dropping thirteen items. The researchers then chose to use a stricter criteria in an effort to shorten the length of the questionnaire and also eliminated items that were highly correlated (and thus too similar). These procedures resulted in a twenty-nine-item questionnaire that was then factor analyzed again to produce the resulting eight factors listed above.[4]

Using the EAT, significant differences were found between low and high EAT scorers on the EDQ total score and six of the eight subscales, indicating some support for the similarity between what is measured on

---

4 To determine the internal reliability, Cronbach's alpha scores were computed for the items on each factor. For seven of the factors, Cronbach's alphas ranged from 0.701 to 0.814. However, for stereotyped behavior, Cronbach's alpha was 0.516. The Cronbach's alpha for the total EDQ score was 0.843. For external validation the EDQ was validated against several other measures.

the EDQ and eating-disordered individuals. However, several differences were also found in the populations suggesting that exercise dependence, as measured by the EDQ, is distinct from the problem of eating disorders. Validation with the Profile of Mood States (POMS) found significant correlations between exercise dependence and depression, anxiety, fatigue, and vigor, suggesting a relationship between exercise dependency and mood disorder. This provides some support for the relationship between exercise dependency and mood. However, many of the correlations were low and, just as with the EAT, the results suggested that the EDQ was not simply a replication of what was measured on the POMS. Thus, there were differences that indicated that exercise was different from either eating disorders or mood disorders, although the authors suggest that the relationship between exercise dependence and eating disorders needs further evaluation.

Building on previous research that sought to identify exercise dependence, Bamber, Cockerill, Rogers, and Carroll (2003) interviewed fifty-six adult female exercisers using the eating disorders examination and the exercise dependence interview. Prior to the semistructured interview, subjects completed the EDQ.[5] Bamber et al. (2003) identified two diagnostic criteria, impairment and withdrawal, from a total of four general dimensions from eleven second-order themes identified through the data input and validated by the third author, Rogers. Impaired functioning was manifested in four areas: psychological, social and occupational, physical, and behavioral. Impairment in at least two areas was necessary for a diagnosis. Withdrawal was present when there was a demonstrated adverse reaction to exercise cessation or an inability to control the amount of exercise. Either criterion was satisfactory for a diagnosis. If an eating disorder accompanied the diagnosed exercise addiction, then the exercise addiction was considered secondary to the eating disorder. If an eating disorder was not present, then the diagnosis was primary exercise dependence.

---

5 Interview data were transcribed and analyzed using nonnumerical unstructured data indexing searching and theorizing (QRS NUD*IST 4.0).

Ten women met the above criteria for exercise dependence, and all ten demonstrated eating-disorder behavior, thus all were secondary exercise dependent. In relation to the EDQ scores and cutoff of higher than 116, all ten scored higher than 116, with a mean of 136.3. The 116 cutoff identified 90% of exercise-dependent individuals, including 10% false positives; a total of 30% of individuals not considered exercise dependent based on Bamber et al.'s (2002) diagnosis tested positive for exercise dependence on the EDQ. Bamber et al. (2003), using both qualitative and quantitative measures, provided clinicians with a tool to diagnose exercise dependence.

This succinct diagnosis outlined in Table 1 is helpful as it is abbreviated and offers a rapid assessment of an individual's proclivity to exercise addiction; however, caution is needed when applying the results of questioning only fifty-six female participants to a much larger and more diverse population of individuals.

Table 1

Primary and Secondary Exercise Dependence

Primary exercise dependence

1. Preoccupation with exercise that has become stereotyped and routine;

2. Significant withdrawal symptoms in the absence of exercise (e.g., mood swings, irritability, insomnia);

3. The preoccupation causes clinically significant distress or impairment in their physical, social, occupational, or other important areas of functioning; and

4. The preoccupation with exercise is not better accounted for by another mental disorder (e.g., as a means of losing weight or controlling calorie intake as in an eating disorder).

Secondary exercise dependence

1. Narrowing of repertoire leading to a stereotyped pattern of exercise with a regular schedule once or more daily;

2. Salience with the individual giving increasing priority over other activities to maintaining the pattern of exercise;

3. Increased tolerance to the amount of exercise performed over the years;

4. Withdrawal symptoms by further exercise;

5. Relief or avoidance of withdrawal symptoms by further exercise;

6. Subjective awareness of a compulsion to exercise; and

7. Rapid reinstatement of the previous pattern of exercise and withdrawal symptoms after a period of abstinence.

Associated features

1. Either the individual continues to exercise despite a serious physical disorder known to be caused, aggravated, or prolonged by exercise and is advised as such by a health professional, or the individual has arguments or difficulties with their partner, family, friends, or occupation.

2. Self-inflicted loss of weight by dieting as a means toward improving performance.

† from "Proposed diagnostic criteria for primary and secondary exercise dependence" by Bamber, Cockerill, Rodgers, & Carroll, 2003, *British Journal of Sports Medicine, 37*, p. 394

Concurrently, Adams, Miller, and Kraus (2003) reviewed the theoretical and diagnostic tools available to the current practicing psychotherapist in the treatment of exercise dependence. They first documented the signs and symptoms of exercise dependence for the purpose of diagnosing behavioral patterns and providing proper treatment. Clinicians were advised to recognize dependence patterns when signs of tolerance, withdrawal, and compulsive behavior appeared in a patient's relationship with exercise. When exercise shifted from being a positively reinforced behavior (people work out to feel the benefits of exercise) to a negatively reinforced behavior (people work out to avoid the effects of withdrawal), exercise addiction was likely present.

Examples of tolerance, withdrawal, and compulsive behavior included exercising for longer and longer durations, moodiness and irritability when missing a workout, and working out despite injury or illness to alleviate the anxiety of missing a workout. Adams et al. (2003) found that those with exercise dependence do not work out to feel good; they work out so that they do not experience the withdrawal effects of not working out. When this is the case, exercise no longer serves as a coping strategy but rather becomes a negatively reinforced behavior and, according to Adams et al., a dependence.

Garman et al. (2004) also excluded committed and elite athletes from their study of 257 undergraduate students, going so far as to eliminate "in-season" collegiate athletes from their sample. Students were evaluated using Davis, Brewer, and Ratusny's (1993) behavioral frequency and psychological commitment to exercise. The students were separated into "obligatory exercisers"—those who followed a regular and structured activity protocol—and "pathological exercisers," for whom social life was compromised for the purposes of physical activity or for whom physical activity compromised the health of the individual. They also differentiated "high" exercisers (those who spent more than six hours per week in physical activity) from "general" exercisers (those who spent fewer than six hours per week in physical activity).

Garman et al. (2004) found that "21.8% of college-age students exercise 360 or more minutes per week and demonstrated at least one exercise dependent response pattern to queries about obligatory or pathological exercise" (p. 221). Dependent-response patterns included feeling anxious or depressed when missing a workout, choosing working out over spending time with friends or family, and working out despite injury or illness. While Garman et al.'s research is an important contribution to the literature concerning exercise dependence, it is limited because they excluded in-season athletes from their study. The overt exclusion of this population in the research concerning exercise dependence demonstrates the lack of research on exercise dependence in collegiate and professional athletes.

Explanations of Exercise Addiction

Thompson and Blanton (1987) offered a biochemical hypothesis for the addictive effects of exercise. In their review article, they outlined the research that has been conducted on the neurochemical pathways in the brain and proposed a catecholamine theory for the "runners high" (Grossman 1985). They referenced the fact that catecholamines (adrenalin and noradrenaline) are secreted during exercise and account for lessening feelings of depression (Morgan 1979). By measuring the release of endogenous opioids in relation to the amount of time an individual exercised, Thoren, Floras, Hoffman, and Seals (1990) found that endogenous opioids and β-endorphins increase a positive mood state and pain threshold in exercisers. The longer a person ran, the more endogenous opioids were released, and the runner felt better and experienced less pain than prior to running.

Davis et al. investigated the relationship between excessive exercise and obsessive compulsiveness in 46 anorexic individuals as compared to 55 individuals who participate in moderate (less than five hours of exercise per week; and 40 high-level exercisers (more than five hours of exercise per week.[6] Davis et al. found that in eating-disorder patients, the amount of physical activity was significantly related to obsessive compulsiveness, weight preoccupation, and "pathological aspects of exercise." In high-level exercisers without eating disorders, only obsessive compulsiveness was significantly related to the amount of physical activity.

6 *Obsessive compulsiveness was measured based on the SCL-90 (Derogatis, 1976), weight preoccupation was measured using the Drive-for-Thinness subscale of the Eating Disorder Inventory (Garner, Olmsted, Bohr, and Garfinkel 1983), and Commitment to Exercise was measured using the Commitment to Exercise Scale (Davis et al. 1993). Using a one-factor ANOVA and pairwise-correlation coefficients,*

According to Davis et al., "Undereating and overexercising become mutually reinforcing behaviors" (1993, p. 967) as both increase the intrasynaptic serotonin (5-hydroxytryptamine) levels in individuals, leading to further obsessive behaviors. The autoaddiction opioid theory (Marrazzi and Luby 1986) refers to the activation of the dopaminergic reward pathway of the brain that is activated by both strenuous exercise and starvation (Aravich, 1996). In other words, individuals become addicted to the chemicals released through starvation and or excessive exercise. Thus while exercise addiction is not its own distinct illness in the DSM, the chemicals released during exercise have a documented addictive potential.

In addition to biological explanations for exercise addiction, Marchant and Levy (2005) looked to sociocultural attitudes of fat phobia to account for the presence of dual symptomology, exercise addiction, and eating pathology. Marchant and Levy measured fat phobia in forty-two exercising individuals (nineteen males; twenty-three females) using the Exercise Dependence Scale (Hausenblas and Downs 2002b) and the Short Form Fat Phobia Questionnaire (Bacon, Scheltema, and Robinson 2001). Through Pearson correlations and Enter Regression method they found that the more one exercised, the more fat phobic one was, and the more anxiety one had around missing a workout. Investigators speculated that exercise addiction may often be associated with body dysmorphia (the misperception of one's body, perceiving oneself as larger than one actually is). While Marchant and Levy studied both male and female athletes, they did not draw conclusions based on the gender of their participants. Rather they looked at the social influences of thin icons as an explanation for the fat-phobic attitudes in excessive exercisers. They too called for further research as to why exercise dependence and fat phobias were mutually reinforcing.

The Documentation of Exercise Addiction

To recap the argument thus far, Morgan contributed to the exercise-addiction literature in 1979 when he likened the exercisers who push themselves to injury to the drug addicts who need more and more of a substance to reach the same high, eventually overdosing. Morgan introduced the notion of tolerance into the discussion, but did not quantify or offer diagnostic criteria concerning exercise tolerance. He merely reported on it through his observations, and in so doing addressed the previously absent topic of "exercise addiction." Next, Sachs and Pargman (1979) discussed the withdrawal effects of exercise addicts, furthering the literature in print concerning exercise addiction. Anshel (1991) continued the conversation of withdrawal effects, further substantiating Sachs and Pargman's claims. Thompson and Blanton (1987) offered a biological explanation for the tolerance and withdrawal effects through their investigation of biochemistry and exercise. Griffiths (1997) broke from the scientific model by presenting a case study. Bamber et al. (2003) continued the conversation concerning the diagnostic criteria and differentiated between primary (its own discrete illness) and secondary exercise addiction (to an eating disorder). Adams et al. (2003) simultaneously proposed similar diagnostic criteria. Terry et al. (2004) added a rapid assessment to the clinician's repertoire of diagnostic tools. Testing these tools against a college-aged population, Garman et al. (2004) investigated the prevalence of exercise addiction in this population. Further testing needs to occur in more specialized populations, athletes in particular. The studies described thus far have not been part of the mainstream psychology literature because psychologists do not recognize exercise as an addiction.

The premise of my work lies in the difficulty of examining the construct of exercise addiction in a competition that requires many of the features proposed to define exercise addiction. To date, exercise addiction is not listed as its own discrete illness in the DSM-IV-TR, nor is there consensus about a single scale for clinicians to assess exercise addiction. Nevertheless, the topic of exercise addiction is present in psychology journals as well as sport studies and medical publications.

Exercise Addiction as Distinct from Eating Disorders

In contrast to the studies described thus far, some researchers (a) distinguish exercise addiction from eating pathology as a "healthier" and distinctly apathological disorder, or (b) laud exercise addiction as a positive coping strategy. To date, there are psychologists who do not believe that exercise addiction is a pathological behavior pattern that warrants diagnostic criteria. In fact, some researchers have gone so far as to argue that not only is exercise addiction benign at best, it is in fact a positive addiction.

Chapman and DeCastro (1990) argued, "Rrunning addiction is associated with positive, not negative psychological characteristics" (p. 289). Thirty-two male and fifteen female runners in the Chapman and DeCastro study completed the Running Addiction Scale, the Commitment to Running Scale (Carmack and Martens 1979), the Personality and Locus of Control Scales (SCL-90-R, Derogatis 1976), Levenson's (1973) Locus of Control Scale, and a questionnaire about running habits (including run frequency and duration). Through correlational analyses, Chapman and DeCastro found the more individuals run, the less depressed, anxious, hostile, paranoid, or obsessive-compulsive they test. Thus they argue that running does increase mood, and can do so without addiction.

Davis and Fox (1993) also found even excessive exercise had a positive psychological affect. They found excessive exercisers (those who exercised at least six times per week for more than one hour per session reported "greater body satisfaction and body focus, were less emotionally reactive (neurotic), and more extraverted than nonexercisers" (p. 201). Three hundred and fifty-one adult women were evaluated on the following subscales: age, body dissatisfaction, body focus, body mass index, percentage body fat, extraversion, and neuroticism. Regression analyses revealed that (a) excessive exercisers differ significantly from nonexcessive exercisers, (b) both excessive exercisers and weight-preoccupied individuals demonstrate a high level of body focus, and (c) weight-preoccupied individuals are more emotionally reactive than excessive exercisers. Davis and Fox thus concluded that excessive exercisers, while sharing some psychological characteristics with weight-conscious individuals, demonstrated higher levels of emotional stability (less reactive) than those who were not excessive exercisers, but were weight preoccupied.

Yates et al. (1983) were among the first to make the connection between male runners and female anorexics. Through their interpretation of unstructured interviews, Yates et al. proposed that because of their running habits, male marathoners were similar to anorexic females in their preoccupation with weight and body fat and adherence to rigid diets, and had an increase in running distances following binging or indiscretions in diet. Yates et al. also noted demographic similarities in family background, socioeconomic status, perfectionism, and depressive tendencies between the sixty interviewed marathoners and anorectic individuals, based on previously published data. Their methodology was problematic as it was based on impressionistic interviews and not standardized measurements, and comparisons were made between male runners and anorexics without a control group.

In a review article, Veale (1987) proposed that exercise dependence is not an extension or mere symptomology of an eating disorder; instead it is its own dependence based on core features of a dependence syndrome outlined by Edwards et al. (1977). Veale offered diagnostic criteria to help sports clinics and psychologists recognize exercise dependence. Veale distinguished exercise addiction from anorexia. "In primary exercise dependence, the exercise is an end in itself and the dieting and weight loss is used to improve performance" (Veale, p. 738). In the case of anorexia and bulimia, the exercise aids in the primary goal of weight loss, and the exercise is only a means to an end—that of losing weight.

In an attempt to empirically evaluate the similarities and differences between anorexics and runners, Blumenthal, O'Toole, and Chang (1984) administered the Minnesota Multiphasic Personality Inventory (Hathaway and McKinley 1948) to forty-three runners and twenty-four patients with anorexia nervosa. The anorectic patients scored more pathological on eight of the ten subscales. While there is a wide range of severity in eating disorders, and anorexia nervosa resides at the more severe end of the continuum, Blumenthal et al. concluded that eating-disorder patients (in their variety of severity) were less psychologically healthy than obligatory runners as defined by the twenty-one-item

Assessment of Obligatory Running (Yates et al. 1983). They concluded then that running is a "healthy" coping strategy, whereas restricted eating is not. Blumenthal et al.'s homogenous assessment of all eating-disorder patients and all obligatory runners is problematic. In contrast to the information presented previously, Blumenthal et al. concluded that individuals who run do not display the same pathology as anorexic individuals and test healthier on the Minnesota Multiphasic Personality Inventory than anorexic patients and thus are not addicts or excessive in their activity.

Nudelman, Rosen, and Leitenberg (1988) also distinguished running from eating disorders in their study that found that men who participate in "high-intensity" running (six or seven runs per week over forty minutes each) were not analogous to women who suffer from bulimia nervosa. An additional male population who exercised less than three to four times per week for twenty to thirty minutes each time were used in this study as a control group. The two male groups completed the Obligatory Running Questionnaire (Blumenthal et al. 1984) and tested significantly different. All three subject groups completed the EAT (Garner and Garfinkel 1979), the Eating Disorders Inventory (EDI; Garner, Olmsted, and Polivy 1983), the Beck Depression Inventory (Beck, Ward, Mendelsohn, and Erbaugh 1961), the Rosenberg Self-esteem Scale (Rosenberg 1979) and the Lawson Social Self-esteem Scale (Lawson, Marshall, and McGrath 1979). One-way ANOVA tested between-group differences and yielded the result that high-intensity male exercisers do not display distorted eating patterns or a preoccupation with food and are not anxious about food consumption. Male runners were statistically equivalent to female bulimics on the Oral Control scale of the EAT. Despite this result, Nudelman et al. deduced that "there is no psychological basis for discouraging men from intense running habits" (p. 633). It is important to note that this research was conducted with only male exercisers, so to extrapolate their conclusions to all runners is problematic. Also, their experimental design crossing genders is somewhat questionable and is not controlled for in their experimental design.

Further research is needed with both a male and female exercise population, particularly because Slay et al. (1998) found that women have a higher incidence of eating pathology than men in association with obligatory running. This means that women who are obligatory runners have a higher likelihood of having an associated eating disorder than men who are obligatory runners. Using a modified version of the Aberdeen Marathon Follow-up Questionnaire (Clough, Shepherd, and Maughan 1990), the Obligatory Runners Questionnaire (Blumenthal et al. 1994) and the EAT (Garner and Garfinkel 1979), Slay et al. surveyed 240 males and eighty-four females from a sample of race participants in a local 4-mile road race and found sixty-three males and twenty-one females qualified as obligatory runners. Using ANOVAs to analyze the data, Slay et al. found obligatory runners scored significantly higher on the EAT and had lower body weight than nonobligatory runners. These effects were stronger in women. Slay et al. hypothesized that perhaps individuals approached running with preexisting pathology. They asserted that running long distances in itself was not a dangerous behavior, but rather the reason people run and the results they hope to achieve through their running could be paramount in explaining the link between running and eating pathology.

In fact, Bamber et al. (2000) asserted that exercise dependence is not a pathology to the extent that it needs to be classified as its own unique (primary) illness. "In the absence of an eating disorder, women identified as being exercise dependent do not exhibit the sorts of personality characteristics and levels of psychological distress that warrant the construction of primary exercise dependence as a widespread pathology" (Bamber et al., 2000). In other words, exercise dependence alone does not warrant its own placement in the DSM-IV, the current text used to diagnose and classify psychological disorders.

Bamber et al. (2000) evaluated their subjects using ten different psychological questionnaires, including the EDQ, the Eating Disorder Examination Self-report Questionnaire, the General Health Questionnaire, the Rosenberg Self-esteem Scale, the Eysenck Personality Questionnaire (Revised), the Body Shape Questionnaire, and the Exercise

Beliefs Questionnaire. Bamber et al. (2000) found that those who scored higher on the EDQ did not exhibit lower levels of general health or lower levels of self-esteem. Subjects who demonstrated eating-disorder pathology did score lower on the General Health Questionnaire and the Self-esteem Scale. Bamber at al. concluded that the presence of exercise dependence did not correlate to eating pathology, and it did not determine ill health physiologically (demonstrated by the General Health Questionnaire) or psychologically (determined by the Self-esteem Scale, the Personality Questionnaire, and the Body Shape Questionnaire). Bamber et al. concluded,

> People identified as being primary exercise dependent show unremarkable levels of psychological morbidity and healthy levels of self-esteem. As such, [Bamber et al.] argue against the notion that primary exercise dependence is a pathology, and certainly undermine the claim that it is a prevalent pathology (2000, p. 130).

Now What?

One of the largest studies to date was conducted by Mond et al. (2006), who sampled 3,472 regularly exercising women ages eighteen to forty-two. Participants completed the Eating Disorder Examination Questionnaire (Fairburn and Beglin 1994), Medical Outcomes Study Short-form Disability Scale[7] (Ware, Kosinski, and Keller 1996), Frequency of Physical Activity, and Commitment to Exercise Scale (Davis et al. 1993). Mond et al. concluded[8] that excessive exercise does exist, but that it is only pathological in conjunction with a primary eating disorder or when feelings of intense guilt accompany the cessation or delay of exercise; however, they caution that in the absence of an eating disorder, excessive exercise is "unlikely to be associated with impairment in psychosocial functioning." Thus, according to Mond et al., excessive exercise,

---

7 7.. *Used to measure quality of life.*

8 *Using the Pearson correlation coefficient and multiple regression models*

while psychologically significant, is only significant in association with an eating disorder.

Adkins and Keel (2005) surveyed 162 female and 103 male undergraduate students who completed the EDI and the Obligatory Exercise Questionnaire as well as questions concerning exercise duration and frequency. They found, through multivariate analysis, disordered eating attitudes and behaviors were positively predicted by Obligatory Exercise Questionnaire scores and negatively predicted by exercise time. Thus they concluded that "excessive exercise," as listed in the DSM-IV under criteria for bulimia nervosa, was actually a misnomer. *Compulsive* exercise, capturing the psychological commitment to exercise, better describes the behavior listed as an associated feature of bulimia nervosa than *excessive*, which alludes to the number of hours spent exercising. Using the Obligatory Exercise Questionnaire and the EDI, Adkins and Keel were able to deduce that it was the quality of the exercise and not the quantity that more accurately described its pathology with the associated eating disorder.

Adkins and Keel's (2005) distinction is important to this work concerning exercise addiction in Ironman athletes, because most of the validated psychological surveys evaluating exercise addiction heavily weight the number of hours spent exercising as a key component of exercise addiction. Ironman athletes spend a great deal of time training; thus the volume of training alone marks Ironman athletes as potential exercise addicts. Adkins and Keel argued that hours alone do not accurately capture the quality of excessive exercise as listed in the DSM-IV as a component of bulimia nervosa.

While the debate continues concerning whether exercise dependence is its own discrete entity, the scales assessing exercise dependence continue to be refined (Bamber, Cockerill, and Carroll 2002; Terry et al. 2004). Exercise addicts are healthier than eating-disorder patients (Blumenthal et al. 1984), and yet display their own unique pathology different from the nonexercise addict (Anshel 1991). Exercise dependence is based on documented withdrawal signs and symptoms (Adams et al. 2003) and tends to be dismissed without an associated pathology of a primary eating disorder (Mond et al. 2006). So what does this mean for the competitive athlete? The debate is ongoing concerning the nature of exercise addiction; however, mental-health practitioners, coaches, and medical doctors alike have been provided with tools—albeit heavily debated ones—to assess the likelihood that an individual suffers from exercise addiction. The obvious exclusion of athletes calls into question the validity of these scales. Division I athletes fall well within the realm of exercise addiction based solely on their rigid practice and competition schedule. The same holds true for the professional athlete and the aspiring Olympian. Existing literature does not take into account high-caliber athletes to detect exercise addiction. There are, however, a few notable studies that address the specific sport of triathlon.

Triathlon-Specific Literature

In January 1996, Virnig and McLeod bridged the gap between the literature on obsessive running and the burgeoning sport of triathlon. Virnig and McLeod found that triathletes had a "slightly healthier" relationship with food than runners. The EAT was administered to 109 runners who competed in a 30 km event and fifty-three triathletes who competed in an international-distance triathlon (1 km swim, 20 km bike, and 6 km run). The authors had three hypotheses: they anticipated that (a) triathletes would have a healthier relationship with food than runners, (b) triathletes and runners would have different motivations for participation, runners for weight loss and triathletes for competition, and (c) triathletes would prefer to train in groups whereas runners would prefer to train alone. These hypotheses were derived from one author's personal involvement in both subcultures and his observations while racing triathlon and running.

Virnig and McLeod (1996) gathered data via questionnaires distributed in prerace packages to potential participants. While the data concerning eating attitudes were analyzed using ANOVA, the other two hypotheses were analyzed descriptively. Qualitative methods such as in-depth interviews were used to elicit a more complete understanding of an athlete's motivation for participation in a sport. The triathletes interviewed were participants in an international-distance triathlon, a triathlon shorter than an Ironman race. Individual motivation for racing is so complex that quantitative measurements do not suffice to properly deduce differences between triathletes and runners. While the data gathered in Virnig and McCleod's study brings triathletes into the conversation concerning exercise addiction, it does so with a limited scope—that of international-distance triathletes alone.

Virnig and McLeod (1996) found that triathletes had healthier eating patterns than runners. Subsequently DiGioacchino DeBate et al. (2002b) probed into the eating patterns of triathletes and found that out of 583 triathlete questionnaires gathered over the World Wide Web in 1999, 28% of females and 11% of males displayed mild distortions of feelings toward food. In other words, close to a third of female triathletes and approximately 10% of male triathletes have less than ideal eating habits and attitudes toward food. In fact, 29% of males and 49% of females reported being "sometimes, or always, terrified about being overweight." Twenty-one percent of males and 47% of females were "sometimes, or always, preoccupied with the desire to be thinner." Twenty-eight percent of males and 43% of females were "sometimes, or always, preoccupied with the thought of having fat on their body" (p. 217). Approximately half of female triathletes and a third of male triathletes were preoccupied with food and bodily appearance. One hundred percent of the subjects in the study reported dissatisfaction with their actual body mass index. Statistics were not compared to a nonathletic population; however, in accordance with previous research (Black 1991; Hauck and Blumenthal 1992; Sundgot-Borgen 1999; Thompson and Sherman, 1993), athletes are more prone to developing eating disorders and demonstrate higher levels of bodily awareness and compulsion compared to their nonathletic counterparts.

DiGioacchino DeBate et al. (2002b) found that 58% of females and 47% of males "were dissatisfied with how they perceive themselves" and

97.3% of female triathletes wished to be smaller than their calculated body mass index. While this research did not address the issue of exercise addiction specifically, it targeted the potential underlying factors leading to exercise addiction—body size dissatisfaction and restricted eating patterns. DiGioacchino DeBate et al. (2002b) commented, "It is also interesting to speculate as to whether the sport attracts athletes with dysfunctional perspective of body size, shape, weight, and food intake patterns, or whether the onset of these problems is a consequence of practicing the sport" (p. 219).

Bell and Howe (1988) asked this question of triathletes. Two hundred forty-nine triathletes who had competed in an Olympic-distance triathlon consisting of a 1-mile swim, 21-mile bike ride, and 6-mile run answered two questionnaires, the Profile of Mood States and a Motivation Rating Scale. Subjects included 160 male and eighty-nine female triathletes, all of whom participated in the same triathlon. The results showed that "successful females had higher psychic vigor, lower tension, and lower total mood disturbance over unsuccessful females, while successful males had lower depression than unsuccessful males" (Bell and Howe, p. 66). The more successful the triathlete, the happier he/she was. This finding offers a potential explanation for compulsive overexercise. The more one exercises, the faster one becomes, and faster individuals will be happier, and competitive athletes are happier when they win.

In Bell and Howe's study (1988), motivating factors for triathlon participation did not vary by gender. The primary reasons triathletes gave for participating in triathlons was for self-improvement, fitness, enjoyment, and competition. Triathletes "scored lower on tension, depression, anger, fatigue, and confusion than elite swimmers and runners but were similar to cyclists" (p. 72). Bell and Howe concluded that "the amount of activity may promote positive mood profiles" and deduced that since triathletes participate in three disciplines, they must be training longer, thus reaping the benefits of the promotion of mood state due to exercise. What these data indicated is that triathletes may, in fact, be "healthier" individuals as demonstrated by increased and more stable mood states than other athletes, a deduction with which Virnig and McLeod (1996) would agree, but with which DiGioacchino DeBate, Wethington, and Sargent (2002a, 2002b) would disagree.

Blaydon and Lindner (2002) most recently administered both the EDQ and the EAT to 203 triathletes, both "age groupers" (recreational triathletes) and professionals. This is the first study of its kind to take into account professional athletes. The investigators found, through clustering methods of data analysis, triathletes can be grouped into four distinct categories. Those who scored high on the EDQ and high on the EAT (high–high), those who scored high on the EDQ and low on the EAT (high–low), those who scored low on the EAT and low on the EDQ (low–low), and those who scored low on the EDQ and high on the EAT (low–high). While investigators found that primary exercise dependence did exist without a corollary eating disorder, the difference between primary and secondary exercise dependence was not statistically significant based on multivariate and mutlifactorial ANOVA. However, the number of professional athletes in the primary exercise-addiction group was high compared to the number of amateur athletes. Also the number of professional athletes who scored high on the EAT was relatively low (although not statistically significant) in relation to their expected distribution. While the researchers did not discuss the differences between professional and amateur athletes other than the above data, the fact that they included and differentiated professional athletes from "age-groupers" is important to the contribution of a more comprehensive account of exercise dependence.

The Triathlon Subculture

The final two studies concerning triathlon look at the triathlon environment as opposed to the individual triathletes. Hilliard (1988) investigated the triathlon culture and found that triathletes were motivated to engage in triathlons for reasons more complex than Bell and Howe (1988) revealed. Hilliard, a triathlete himself, observed and participated in nine triathlons ranging from sprint to Olympic distance. He observed three other sprint or Olympic distance races and, based on extensive field notes and interviews with participants, drew his conclusions. Unlike many of the previous investigations, this study did not use quantitative measures, but rather the researcher reflected on his own participation and engaged in extensive dialogue with fellow competitors.

According to Hilliard (1988), triathlon popularity in the 1980s stemmed from reasons beyond health, fitness, fun, and competition. He asserted that the allure of triathlon actually arose from athletes' search for control in their life. When work, family, and "the rest of life" seemed unsatisfying and out of control, individuals flocked to triathlons to assert control over something, in this case their body.

> [Triathlon] provides participants with an opportunity to put themselves on the line, that is, to take risks, control the action, and take credit for accomplishment. The need to feel this kind of action may be presumed to be especially strong among the young and highly educated, who are socialized to believe that their careers will offer them such opportunities but who frequently find themselves mired in the middle levels of corporate structures (Hilliard, 1988, p. 312).

Triathlon offers an opportunity to feel embodied and self-satisfied in a corporate climate devoid of reward other than the monetary kind.

Hilliard (1988) asserted that triathlon is its own subculture, complete with its own language (gels, gu's, T1, T2, PR, HR, LT, and other abbreviations only fellow triathletes might recognize), its own set of equipment (wet suits, bikes, and high-tech running shoes and gear), and its own racing scene. The subculture does not dissolve when races end; instead there are complex networks of training clubs, periodicals devoted to triathlon, and now Internet Web sites. Hilliard contended that the body-marking process, when an athlete's number is written on both arms and both legs (in order to identify athletes while they are swimming, biking, and running), "marks the transition from identity based on dominant statuses to identity as a triathlete" (Hilliard, p. 307). This unique identity further cements an entry into a distinct subculture. Hilliard articulately described the triathlete experience from an insider perspective. He commented that "triathlon competition is a cyclical process; for the committed triathlete, the end of one race marks the beginning of planning and preparation for the next" (p. 309). Thus Hilliard not only documents the salience of triathlon as a distinct component to identity, but he also documents the "cyclical" and potentially obsessive nature of triathlon.

Another insider investigation of triathlon subculture was conducted by Granskog (1992), a Southern California triathlete who focused on the unique identity of triathletes. She looked at the ways in which gender were enacted and redefined in Southern California triathlon training groups. She noted (from her own experience) that female triathletes who trained in the company of men often are respected as competitive equals in the realm of triathlon. While Granskog outlined the multiple varieties of training networks, including swimming, running, cycling, triathlon, single sex, and mixed sex, she focused on the mixed arenas of training and racing and deduced that "the cooperative sharing that takes place among both men and women during training provides both genders with an opportunity to transcend traditional gender expectations" (p. 88). Granskog concluded that "the triathlete life-style thus represents the creation of a new cultural reality, one that reflects the transformation of gender roles taking place within our society today" (p. 90). Granskog's work is contextualized within her own experience and was influenced by this experience. One example is her incidental remark that "triathletes value themselves for their balanced approach to overall fitness" (p. 79). Granskog did not indicate from where she drew this conclusion. Instead, she celebrates the "transcendence" of women into the triathlon realm. In so doing, Granskog demonstrates the very misunderstanding that Bordo (1997) and Duncan (1994) caution against. When participation is in the service of an aesthetic, ideal female liberation is thwarted rather than actualized.

Ironman athletes are complex individuals, minds, bodies, gendered beings, who exist in a socially constructed sphere. Their meaning and value are defined by the current climate they inhabit. To understand this climate and the associated meaning of the Ironman body, I presented the gendered climate of the sporting realm to situate the legacy of masculinity in the sporting realm. I presented the insights of postmodern gender theory to delineate the ways in which gendered beings are constructed in society, Ironman and non-Ironman athletes alike. And finally, I presented the psychological literature concerning exercise dependence and addiction to fully explore the contested construct and its potential use in describing the behavioral patterns and psychological profiles of some Ironman athletes.

Thus the purpose of this literature review was to present the history of women in sport as a highly gendered space, the insights offered by postmodern theory (bodies are a social construct), and the contested construct of exercise dependence and addiction in the field of psychology, all of which I draw upon to tell the story of Ironman athletes. These triathletes are gendered subjects who have been excluded from sport, they are discursive subjects who may be influenced by a thin social aesthetic, and they are potentially pathological subjects who may demonstrate signs of exercise dependence.

Chapter 3: From the Field

The research presented here was gathered as a mixed-method exploratory design using both qualitative data gathered in interviews at Ironman race sites from 2003 to 2005 and quantitative data collected from an online survey administered from June 2006 through October 2006 to examine the prevalence of exercise addiction in the specific population of Ironman triathletes and the extent to which social attitudes about gender-appropriate appearance influence Ironman athletes. The quantitative aspect of the study comprises the EDQ and the SATAQ 3-R to determine the percentage of Ironman athletes who demonstrate warning signs for exercise dependence and to evaluate the extent to which social attitudes toward gender-appropriate appearance influence male and female Ironman athletes.

The specific exploratory design used in this study was the instrumental development/selection model (see Figure 1). Qualitative research was first conducted to examine trends, topics of interest, and emergent themes amongst the population under investigation, namely Ironman athletes. From the themes that emerged through interview data collection and examination, I selected existing instruments to further investigate the qualitative themes, in accordance with the exploratory design method. Once the interviews were transcribed and coded for themes, a survey was used to quantify the prevalence of the themes observed through qualitative data gathering. Using both quantitative and qualitative data creates a more nuanced and accurate picture of the Ironman community. In this design the researcher qualitatively explores the research topic with a small group of participants to demonstrate the need for the quantitative instruments. Researchers using this design often emphasize the quantitative aspect of the study.

In summary, the exploratory mixed-method approach allowed for the gathering and synthesizing of both qualitative and quantitative data in a linear fashion so that the qualitative data-gathering informed the further investigation quantitatively. The results not only create a rich qualitative and quantitative picture of the Ironman triathlete but also offer a detailed analysis of the existence and prevalence of exercise addiction in this highly specified community of athletes.

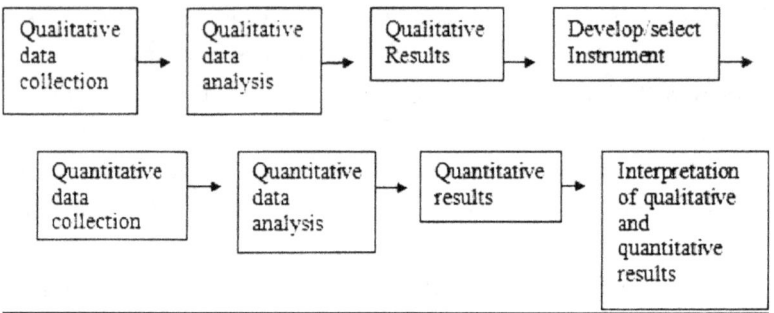

Figure 1. Exploratory design: instrument development/selection model.
From *Designing and conducting mixed methods research* by J. Creswell and V. Plano Clark, 2007, p. 76.

Findings

Specifically, five questions guided this mixed-method exploratory design study. Two questions were qualitative in nature, two were quantitative, and one combined both qualitative and quantitative findings. I present my findings here organized according to the question that guided the gathering of data. So to address the first research question concerning the qualities of exercise dependence described in an interview setting, Ironman athletes were interviewed and four themes emerged from the data: Ironman as a salient component of *identity*, Ironman as a unique *mentality*, Ironman as an *obsession*, and Ironman as an *extreme challenge*.

Ironman Identity

Ironman is not just a race for these athletes; it is integral to their sense of self. CL described how influential Ironman training is for her:

It becomes so much a way of life, so this is what I am about, this is what I do. I wake up in the morning and the first thing I think about is going out and training, and if I don't get to do that, it's a huge part of my day; I feel incomplete. So I can't really begin the day without it.

Ironman training shapes CL's daily existence, without which she would feel lost. Ironman is not only a race; it is an all-encompassing attribute for many of these racers as well. "It's my life…it completes me" (CL). LL also described Ironman as his life: "It's been my life for the last fifteen years." Both CL and LL are professional athletes, so Ironman training and racing is not only a central component of their day; it is also their livelihood.

ND, another professional triathlete who is married to a professional triathlete, talked about Ironman as a way of life. "I was definitely not born to do this. It's not my calling. But it's a beautiful way to live. The healthiest lifestyle I can imagine." ND and her husband are both successful triathletes and are able to make a living through their racing.

Nonprofessional triathletes also referred to Ironman racing and training as a way of life. NY, a very successful older triathlete, commented, "It's great for morale and confidence and lifestyle and everything, and I think it's just a good way to live." Age groupers also derive a sense of self from their Ironman racing. KD, a mother and a successful attorney, viewed her Ironman racing and training as "just mine; it's selfish but it feels good." Ironman is her time for herself: when other identities of motherhood, lawyer, and wife describe her in relation to another being, Ironman describes her in relation to herself. She deemed this selfish, but she also puts a positive spin on the word "selfish," indicating the benefit she derives from it. A total of ten athletes, as shown in Table 2 (59%), mentioned how influential the Ironman identity is to their sense of self. Their identity and subjectivity, albeit malleable, are predicated on their participation in Ironman races. They purposefully shape their body through training and take pride in their accomplishments as Ironman competitors. Their subjectivity is substantiated by their Ironman finishes, but their bodies alone do not capture their complete Ironman identity.

Ironman Mentality

While the Ironman body is consciously crafted through training, Ironman racing requires a distinct mental fortitude. When asked if a certain body type is better suited for Ironman competition, ten athletes countered with the opinion that Ironman competition and success are dictated more by a strong and focused mental game than a perfectly crafted physique. TB, a very successful professional male triathlete, stated, "Without the mind, the body is nothing. You need to be mentally trained. You need mental strength for the Ironman." He knows intimately what it takes to win Ironman competitions as he has won (and lost) many in his career. Evaluating the successes and failures of his racing résumé has led him to the belief that mental fortitude wins and loses races, not genetics, biology, or training alone.

CL, a professional female Ironman athlete, reiterated TB's insight. "You can train the body to a certain point, but your mind actually takes over when physically you can't go any further; you can convince yourself you can actually do a lot more." Races are won and lost through this "Ironman mentality," and professionals are not the only ones who commented on this phenomenon.

A burgeoning female age-group triathlete, RL, also spoke of the Ironman mentality and what it takes to complete races. "When your mind gives in, it's over. So whether your body feels okay or not, when you're mind gives up you're done." The mind is central to completion, according to RL. The Ironman mentality gets an athlete across the finish line, according to RL. PA, another female age-grouper, concurred. "Ironman is on the inside, not in the body. Ironman is a mind." Using postmodern feminist theory to understand how athletes describe their identity, Ironman athletes articulate how their body is constructed through their mental fortitude. Their ability to complete a race resides in their mind, which in turns spurs the body on to accomplish seemingly insurmountable feats. Postmodern feminist theory, and Grosz (1994) and Butler (1990) in particular, theorize about the creation of the body through the mind. Ironman athletes demonstrate this theory through the articulation and understanding of their Ironman subjectivity, comprising both their mentality and their physicality.

Ironman is not only an identity; it is a mind, a mentality, and a central component to success. Professionals and age groupers alike voiced this insight in interviews. Female age grouper CN concluded, "There isn't an Ironman body type, there is an Ironman mentality." Ten athletes (59%) spoke about the distinct Ironman mind and the mental fortitude the race dictates and demands.

Obsession

Digging deeper into this Ironman mind, athletes describe the obsession of Ironman racing. A number of athletes I interviewed admitted that Ironman could become obsessive. Athletes did not identify themselves as obsessive, but instead pointed to the potential in the Ironman community. According to RL, "If you look around at the type of person that's involved in this sport, everyone is a…there's a particular type of person that is crazy enough to do this sort of stuff."

So while Ironman athletes spoke of Ironman racing as an identity, and more specifically a strong and determined mentality, they also acknowledged the potential pitfall for this encompassing identity and strong-willed mentality to work against them, to turn what they view as a positive attribute into a negative one. JP, a female age-group triathlete, without implicating herself, said, "Ironman could be healthy; it could also get obsessive. Fitness has nothing to do with health." Admitting that Ironman athletes are fit (in order to accomplish the goal of completing the race, one must be fit), she conceded this point, but was careful to disentangle the notion of fitness from the notion of health. She clearly articulated they are not the same, and that one can be fit and unhealthy simultaneously.

JP alludes to the concepts outlined by Bordo (1989, 1993, 1997), Cole (1993), and Duncan (1994) that even though female athletes are strong, they may also be disempowered if their "strength" comes from their extreme dieting and exercise in the pursuit of a thin aesthetic. JG, a highly successful female age grouper, reiterated JP's point, stating, "Ironman is healthy, but it can also get obsessive." Ironman *could* be healthy, but it is not necessarily always healthy. Here JG asserted that Ironman *is* healthy.

While JG was assertive in her declarative statement, KD questioned the long-term effects of Ironman and disagreed with JG, stating, "It is not all that healthy." RL too juxtaposed JG's emphatic affirmation by using the word "crazy" to describe the hour at which her Ironman boyfriend and his brother (both professional triathletes) awoke to begin their training day. "I was living with him and his brother and they were getting up at *crazy* hours every morning and training, so I decided the least I could do was go along for a ride." After repeatedly joining her boyfriend and his brother at this "crazy" hour of the morning on rides, she took to the lifestyle and became an Ironman athlete herself.

One of the first topics that athletes spoke about was the Ironman lifestyle as integral to their identity. They then relayed the specifics of that identity in relation to the mental fortitude necessary for finishing an Ironman race. Third, they expanded on the identity and mentality and acknowledged the need for balance as Ironman racing, as an identity and mentality, has the potential to become all encompassing. Female age grouper CN said, "Ironman can get obsessive and take over someone's life." WI offered a solution to the obsessive potential in her statement, "Ironman is a healthy lifestyle, that is, if you can balance it all" (she said this final clause laughing—as though balancing is perhaps impossible). According to the athletes I interviewed, Ironman is a lifestyle both in the positive and potentially negative sense of the word, and balance seems to be the secret to keeping Ironman a positive side of their lives. A total of seven of the seventeen athletes interviewed acknowledged the potential for "obsession" in the sport of Ironman triathlon and identified the possibility that Ironman is not actually a healthy endeavor. Ironman athletes allude to the phenomenon that Ironman athletes are potential exercise addicts. Qualitative data confirmed this theory, and quantitative data tested its prevalence.

Ultimate Challenge

The final theme that emerged from the interview data concerning exercise addiction focused more on the race itself and less on the identity and attributes of those who race. In describing the Ironman race, male age-grouper BU commented, "It is the ultimate physical and mental test in a one-day endurance event." Returning again to the Ironman mentality, BU brought the conversation full circle when he described the Ironman both as a physical and mental race. RL too described the race as a physical and mental challenge. "There are very few things that push your body and your mind and your whole person to do something like that. Definitely it's extreme and definitely it pushes you. It's an extreme challenge." While RL stated that Ironman is extreme, she qualified her use of the word *extreme* with her addendum to the comment, "It is an extreme challenge."

Why do Ironman athletes race? Because it is a challenge, because it is extreme, and, according to female age grouper CN, "I race Ironman because it's there; it's a personal goal for me." After years of competing in shorter-distance triathlons, CN felt she had to try her hand at the Ironman race.

While RL's boyfriend and his crazy training hours initially introduced her to the Ironman way of life, she races for no one but herself. RL stated, "I'm going out there to prove to myself that I can do this." The extreme challenge is a testament to the mental fortitude of RL and gives her a sense of self. Her story captures the common sentiment among the athletes interviewed. A total of six athletes (35%) described the extreme challenge of the Ironman event, again, alluding to the potentially obsessive and extreme nature of Ironman, thus drawing (or creating) a disproportionate number of exercise addicts.

In summary, four themes emerged from the data: Ironman as a salient component of *identity*, Ironman as a unique *mentality*, Ironman as an *obsession*, and Ironman as an *extreme challenge*. These four themes aptly highlight the salient qualities of Ironman athletes, both positive and negative. While Ironman athletes acknowledged that Ironman is central to their identity and recognized their "unique" mentality, they also identified Ironman as potentially obsessive. They are proud of their ability to take on the extreme challenge of Ironman racing while simultaneously cautious of its potential for ill health manifested in the form of obsession. Thus, in an interview setting, Ironman athletes discussed the extreme challenge of the race, the mental fortitude it takes to complete the race, the sense of identity they derive from accomplishing the challenge they set out before themselves, and the potential that the challenge and the commitment to accomplishing that challenge has to become obsessive. The carefully constructed identity reflects the postmodern amalgamation of mind and body, producing the cultural artifact of the Ironman subjectivity. Their identity arises from their mind, their body, their mentality, their training regime, and culminates in their corporeality. Their unique subjectivity alludes to the potential pitfalls of this very dedicated and carefully constructed comportment.

While the four emergent categories from the interview data do not align perfectly with the DSM-IV's definition of dependence, the fact that Ironman athletes willingly acknowledged and articulated the potential for, in their own words, "obsession" is an important contribution to the conversation surrounding exercise addiction and its specific application with particular subpopulations of athletes, in this case Ironman athletes. The literature reviewed has not shown the themes of identity, mentality, and extreme challenge. This may be something that is unique to the Ironman event.

In the existing literature, obsession has been documented in endurance runners (Yates et al. 1983). Bamber et al. (2003) defined primary exercise dependence as a "preoccupation" with exercise. Subjects who identified that Ironman racing and Ironman training has the potential to become "obsessive" highlight the potential for exercise addiction in the community of Ironman athletes.

Identity has also been noted as a salient theme in the exercise addiction research. Sachs and Pargman (1979) classified exercise addicts as those who found exercise "integral" to their existence. Ironman athletes identified their training and racing as a salient component of their identity, thus qualifying themselves as exercise addicts according to Sachs and Pargman. Terry et al. (2004) asserted, "Addicted exercisers view exercise as the central part of their lives" (p. 490). When Ironman athletes spoke about Ironman as a salient component of their identity, they were simultaneously labeling themselves, according to the definition offered by Terry et al., as exercise addicts. Thus two themes identified by Ironman triathletes corroborate existing literature concerning exercise dependence and offer warning signs of dependence patterns that exist among Ironman triathletes.

Quantitative Findings

The following section answers the second question guiding this project: to what extent do Ironman athletes demonstrate high levels of exercise dependence on the Exercise Dependence Questionnaire? The EDQ consists of a total score and eight subscales. The eight subscales include interference with social/family/work life, positive reward, withdrawal symptoms, exercise for weight control, insight into problem, exercise for social reasons, exercise for health reasons, and stereotyped behavior.

Table 4 shows the mean score for the total EDQ for both males (110) and females (101.6). The standard deviation represents the variability in the responses. Males and females did not score significantly differently from one another in any portion of the EDQ; thus it can be concluded that Ironman athletes, male and female, did not differ significantly on the EDQ due to gender.[9]

9 *Male and female Ironman athletes scored higher than Zmijewski and Howard's (2003) controls (males= $t(132) = 4.2, p < .05$, females=$t(138) = 3.9, p < .05$). All inferential statistics were checked to ensure there was no violation of the homogeneity of variance*

Nine out of twenty-seven males (33%) were above the cutoff score for exercise dependence of 116 mentioned by Bamber et al. (2003), and four out of thirteen females (23%) met these criteria, thus scoring in the "pathological" range for exercise addiction.

Male and female Ironman athletes scored significantly higher than controls in total EDQ scores. They also scored higher than controls in the following subscales: interference with social/work/family life, positive reward, insight into problem, exercise for social reasons, and exercise for health reasons. Males scored higher than controls in exercise for weight control. Neither the females nor the males were significantly different from the controls on withdrawal symptoms, however females also were not statistically different for exercise for weight control as compared to the controls.

Female Ironman athletes scored higher than eating-disorder patients in interference with social/work/family life, insight into problem, exercise for social reasons, and stereotyped behavior. Female Ironman athletes scored lower than eating-disorder patients in the following categories: positive reward and exercise for health reasons. Female Ironman athletes did not significantly differ from eating-disorder patients in total EDQ scores, withdrawal symptoms, and exercise for weight control.

EDQ Scores

	Current Project (n = 40: 27 M, 13 F)		Controls† (n = 234: 121 M, 113 F)		Exercise Dependent†† (n = 43)		Eating Disorder†† (n = 14)	
	Mean	S.D.	Mean	S.D.	Mean	S.D.	Mean	S.D.
Total EDQ Scores								
Males	110	15.2	89.6 *	22.7	NA	NA	NA	NA
Females	101.6	19.4	91.3 *	20.9	129.7 *	14.1	97.0	15.5
Interference social/work/family								
Males	21.9	5.83	10.9 *	5.2	NA	NA	NA	NA
Females	21.2	4.9	9.7 *	4.9	18.3 *	6.4	10.1 *	3.8
Positive reward								
Males	8.2	3.1	18.1 *	6.2**	NA	NA	NA	NA
Females	7.4	3.9	19.1 *	5.5**	22.1 *	3.5	20.2 *	5.0
Withdrawal symptoms								
Males	12.7	4.1	11.7	4.9	NA	NA	NA	NA
Females	10.5	4.8	12.0	5.5	5.7 *	3.7	12.5	5.4
Exercise for weight control								
Males	16.8	4.0	12.4 *	4.8	NA	NA	NA	NA
Females	14.6	4.1	14.1	5.4**	17.3	4.2	17.3	4.8
Insight into problem								
Males	21.6	2.8	7.2 *	4.2**	NA	NA	NA	NA
Females	21.1	3.9	6.3 *	3.2	8.6 *	4.7	7.1 *	6.2
Exercise for social reasons								
Males	13.4	3.1	6.8 *	3.4	NA	NA	NA	NA
Females	12.8	3.1	6.1 *	3.0	11.7	3.7	7.6 *	3.2
Exercise for health reasons								
Males	5.8	2.2	14.7 *	3.7**	NA	NA	NA	NA
Females	6.0	2.0	16.0 *	3.8**	18.4 *	10.6**	15.8 *	3.7**
Stereotyped behavior								
Males	9.7	2.2	7.9	3.6	NA	NA	NA	NA
Females	8.1	2.8	7.5	3.2	10.7 *	2.9	5.7 *	2.6

Note. $*p = < .05$

**FMax test significant for potential violations of homogeneity of variance

† Source: "Exercise dependence and attitudes toward eating in young adults" by Zmijewski & Howard, 2003, *Eating Behaviors, 4,* p. 186.

†† Source: "The pathological status of exercise dependence" by Bamber, Cockerill, & Carroll, 2000, *British Journal of Sports Medicine, 34,* p. 128.

In additional analyses, Spearman Rho correlations were performed to examine how responses on various subscales related to responses on other subscales for both males and females. Table 5 presents the results with females above the major diagonal and males below.

The statistically significant findings for females included positive reward and withdrawal (p = .86, $p < .001$) and exercise weight and insight (p = .61, $p < .03$). In other words, females who exercised for positive reward reasons were more likely to experience withdrawal symptoms. Females who had more insight were more likely to exercise for weight reasons.

Table 5

Spearman Rho Correlations and p-Values for Females and Males on the Total EDQ and Subscales.

Females / Males	Total EDQ	Interference	Positive reward	Withdrawal	Exercise-weight	Insight	Exercise-social	Exercise-health	Stereotyped behavior
Total EDQ		.37 (.21)	.91 (.001)*	.83 (.001)*	.69 (.01)*	.50 (.08)	.41 (.16)	.23 (.45)	.52 (.07)
Interference	.64 (.001)*		.08 (.80)	.14 (.65)	.21 (.49)	.41 (.17)	.33 (.27)	-.15 (.63)	-.19 (.54)
Positive reward	.33 (.09)	-.17 (.39)		.86 (.001)*	.54 (.06)	.42 (.15)	.27 (.38)	.25 (.42)	.51 (.07)
Withdrawal	.65 (.001)*	.24 (.23)	.42 (.03)*		.47 (.10)	.49 (.09)	.32 (.29)	.13 (.68)	.38 (.20)
Exercise-weight	.69 (.001)*	.27 (.18)	.23 (.24)	.39 (.045)*		.61 (.03)*	.13 (.66)	-.15 (.62)	.15 (.62)
Insight	.40 (.04)*	.42 (.03)*	.11 (.60)	-.06 (.79)	.13 (.52)		.22 (.47)	-.25 (.41)	-.10 (.75)
Exercise-social	.61 (.001)*	.16 (.43)	.24 (.23)	.58 (.002)*	.29 (.14)	.09 (.65)		.15 (.63)	-.04 (.90)
Exercise-health	.48 (.01)*	.29 (.15)	.19 (.33)	.04 (.84)	.40 (.04)*	.38 (.052)	.13 (.51)		.67 (.01)*
Stereotyped behavior	.39 (.048)*	.10 (.63)	.18 (.36)	.12 (.57)	.29 (.15)	.28 (.16)	.13 (.51)	.42 (.03)*	

* indicates significant correlation ($p < .05$)

A description of the statistically significant findings for males is outlined below. For interference and insight into problem ($\rho = .42, p < .03$), males who claimed that exercise interferes with their social/family/work life were more likely to score higher on the insight into problem subscale. The relationship between withdrawal symptoms and positive reward ($\rho = .42, p < .03$) is also statistically significant, suggesting that males who exercised for positive reward reasons were more likely to experience withdrawal symptoms.

For exercise for weight reasons ($\rho = .39, p < .05$) and exercise for social reasons ($\rho = .58, p < .002$), males who experienced withdrawal symptoms were more likely to exercise for positive reward, weight, and social reasons. For exercise for weight reasons and exercise for health reasons ($\rho = .40, p < .04$), males who exercised for weight reasons also tended to exercise for health reasons. For exercise for health reasons and stereotyped behavior ($\rho = .42, p < .03$), males who exercised for health reasons tended to have a more repetitive workout routine.

In summary, comparing control subjects with Ironman males and females reported significantly higher total EDQ scores, thus demonstrating higher levels of exercise dependence. Males and females scored significantly higher on the subscales interference with social/work/family, positive reward, insight into problem, exercise for social reasons, and exercise for health reasons than control subjects. Males tested significantly higher than controls in exercise for weight control, and females did not.

Females demonstrated higher levels of exercise dependence than exercise-dependent individuals in the following subcategories of the EDQ: interference with social/work/family, positive reward, withdrawal symptoms, insight into problem, exercise for health reasons, and stereotyped behavior. Female Ironman athletes demonstrated higher levels of exercise dependence in comparison with eating-disorder patients in the following categories: interference with social/work/family, positive reward, insight into problem, exercise for social reasons, exercise for health reasons, and stereotyped behavior.

Results showed that both male and female Ironman athletes who exercise for positive reward are more likely to experience withdrawal symptoms if exercise is removed from their daily routine. Females who reported more insight into their problem are more likely to exercise for weight reasons. Males who claimed that exercise interferes with their social/family/work life are more likely to score higher on the insight into problem subscale, and males who experience withdrawal symptoms are more likely to exercise for positive reward, weight, and social reasons. Thus, Ironman athletes exhibited more exercise dependence than the control population. Although the exercise-dependent individuals have significantly higher overall scores than female Ironman athletes, on the subscales of the EDQ female Ironman athletes show more exercise dependence than exercise-dependent individuals. Female Ironman athletes score significantly higher on interference, withdrawal, and insight into problem, and they experience less positive reward from their efforts. Female Ironman athletes do not test significantly different from eating-disorder patients and report higher levels of interference, insight into problem, exercise for social reasons, and stereotyped behavior. Female Ironman athletes also report less positive reward from their efforts. (Data were not available to compare male Ironman athletes to exercise-dependent and eating-disorder populations.)

While Terry et al. (2004) asserted exercise addicts were highly motivated by intrinsic rewards, results in this study challenge their assertion. Both male and female Ironman athletes reported lower positive reward scores than controls. Research that touts exercise as a positive addiction (Chapman and DeCastro 1990; Davis and Fox 1993) is challenged by this finding that Ironman athletes, in fact, are not motivated by positive rewards. They do however score very high on withdrawal scales, supporting the theory that exercise dependence is a negative rather than a positive addiction.

Morgan (1979), Sachs and Pargman (1979), Anshel (1991), Morris et al. (1990), and Terry et al. (2004) identified withdrawal as a strong sign of exercise dependence. Ironman athletes in this study scored higher on the withdrawal subscale than documented exercise addicts thus demonstrating that Ironman athletes demonstrate very high levels of exercise dependence according to the current literature and diagnostic tools used to determine exercise dependence.

Further examination reveals that while Sachs and Pargman (1979) defined the running addict as an individual who exercised six to seven days per week for one hour or more, in the quantitative sample all of the Ironman athletes, those in this study exercised more than seven hours per week, and yet all did not test pathological on the EDQ. The average time spent exercising was reported to be 16.43 hours per week, with the highest training volume at thirty hours and the lowest at eight hours per week. Garman et al. (2004) also classified "obligatory exercisers" as any subjects that followed a regular exercise program, which again would include all of the Ironman athletes in this study.

Thus, while current research on exercise dependence using exercise frequency and duration as positive signs for dependence implicates all Ironman athletes as exercise dependent, this study's result indicates otherwise. Not all Ironman athletes scored in the pathological range on the EDQ. Nine out of twenty-seven males (33%) were above the cutoff score for exercise dependence of 116 as mentioned by Bamber et al. (2003), and four out of thirteen females (23%) met these criteria. Thus caution must be used when adopting exercise time and frequency as signs of exercise addiction.

Social Attitudes Towards Appearance

While earlier reports of interview data addressed the body and identity of Ironman athletes, this line of questioning probed deeper into the motivations for participation in Ironman racing by inquiring about the similarities and differences between a social aesthetic and an ideal Ironman body type. I attempted to unpack motivation by asking informants to either corroborate with or challenge the notion that Ironman racing was in service of a patriarchal ideal of beauty. If informants identified that Ironman bodies and idealized beauty stood in opposition to one another, then deductively Ironman racing is not a means to obtaining an idealized image of beauty. If, however, Ironman bodies and idealized beauty align, motivation to race becomes more complex, and Ironman could be the means to obtaining an end, or the end itself; thus the motivation becomes less clear.

When asked the question "Is there an Ironman body type?" five athletes answered *yes*, there is a distinct Ironman body type. All were female respondents. ND explained,

> There are some body trends among the best women in our sport. That is, for Ironman racing. The top five or ten women in the world are pretty damn lean (which can sometimes equate to being too skinny), usually small (not very tall and lanky), often more of a runner's build (thin legs, less muscle mass in the legs, but very ripped). Ironman triathletes in general are pretty well-rounded; they just seem to have more muscle tone than most athletes.

JG concurred: "Ironman bodies are more balanced. They are stronger overall compared to skinny runners and bikers with huge legs." Because the Ironman combines three distinct sports these athletes believed that Ironman bodies are a conglomeration of the swimmer type, the cyclist build, and the runner to produce a more well-rounded Ironman athlete.

While these athletes identified a trend in Ironman bodies, other athletes believed that Ironman bodies come in all shapes and sizes. A total of eight athletes believed there is not an Ironman body type. Only one male answered this question; however, all quotations presented here are from female respondents.

When asked if there was an Ironman body type, CN held out her arms (while standing in just a purple bathing suit) and declared, "This is it." She explained, "There is not an Ironman body type; there is an Ironman mentality." PA reiterated, "Ironman is on the inside, not in the body. Ironman is a mind;, any size body can do it." Because any size body can do it, Ironman can be considered empowering as the focus here, in the athletes own words, is the accomplishment and not the appearance of the athlete.

Eight athletes, all female respondents, believed that the Ironman body type does not correlate with the ideal cultural aesthetic. ND parsed the difference between ideal bodies within and outside of the Ironman. She commented, "I think we get mixed messages. It really depends where you look. In the magazines, beauty is about being really skinny and having a perfect complexion. At sporting events, beauty is about being strong and taking care of yourself," conclusively locating agency in the action and not in the pursuit of an aesthetic ideal. RL continued ND's line of thought with the following assertion:

You know, I think triathlon does a huge amount for your ego and your self-confidence, and it's the one sport where it doesn't matter what you look like, and it doesn't matter how you do, and it doesn't matter whether you fall over on the side of the road or not. Everyone is very supportive and there for you, and it does a huge amount. I think if more young girls got into it, there would be so much less problem, problems with image and eating and all of those ridiculous things. Because it does. You get to a point where you actually realize, it doesn't matter what I look like, doesn't matter how I behave, everyone is equal out there. Which is really nice. Huh?

NC explained that Ironman athletes are "healthy women, not Barbie dolls." KD agreed with NC in the first part of her statement that Ironman athletes are healthier than the standards of beauty for women in the United States; however, she contradicted herself in the latter part of her statement: "Standards of beauty for women are not as healthy as Ironman bodies, but Ironman bodies are very thin, but muscular as well. The Ironman body type makes me think of gaunt faces, but this isn't healthy." As KD found herself describing Ironman bodies, she realized the inherent contradiction in what she was saying and worked through the tension of what it means to be healthy, fast, and pretty.

Four athletes believed that Ironman body types and cultural images of beauty align (again, all responses were from female athletes). ND stated, "I think people appreciate Ironman bodies in the same way they appreciate the bodies of supermodels."

NY explained,

If you train, you are going to be fit. You know, it just sort of happens, the type happens naturally from working out....A fit body is more attractive than an unfit body and I think that's where the body is supposed to be. I mean, you don't have to be super, super muscular, but there is a...I do think it's nice to be fit and strong and whatever, especially when you're older. It makes a difference in how you feel. Stay fit, stay muscular, you can feel it in your body, if you are not in good shape or if you are, and I think that affects the attitude and I think you look better if you feel good about yourself.

Her cultural aesthetic is the Ironman aesthetic, which, according to her, happens naturally through training. She shifts agency from the act to the appearance and then back to the act itself. In so doing, she mirrors the movement of identity from the external to the internal to the external once again, exactly as Butler (1993) theorizes.

Gender Equity

Although women in the Ironman racing realm are not immune to the social pressures to conform to a cultural aesthetic, they are able to shift the focus from what they look like to what they can accomplish with their bodies. For the female triathlete, Ironman is potentially empowering. Most feel it does not matter what someone looks like; what matters is what he/she is able to do with his/her body, with his/her mind, and with his/her heart. This athletic venue takes the attention off appearance and places it on accomplishment instead. For a female immersed in a body-conscious culture, Ironman is empowering. And twelve athletes believed that women are respected in the Ironman racing realm.

RL related, "Everyone has this huge amount, either whether you're an athlete or whether you're a supporter, have an amazing amount of respect for the fact that you're out there doing it. That's what counts." Accomplishment is lauded over appearance. Ironman athletes, while competing, stray from the rigid definition of beauty and demonstrate their inner beauty—the strength of their minds and their hearts to complete the daunting task of the Ironman triathlon. RL was not the only one to comment on the respect that women athletes receive while racing.

ND commented that diversion from appearance to accomplishment is empowering for women and is a hallmark for the gender-inclusive nature of the Ironman race. She said,

> I think women triathletes are completely respected. We're as tough as the dudes. Triathlete guys are blown away by us. We're not being all pretty out there. We blow snot, we pee on our bikes, we barf on the side of the road. We're all in the same boat. I like the chance to let it all hang out on the playing field. I love beating the guys. I love that we get to race against the men…. Women gut it out like the guys and so women are respected by women and by men in Ironman.

Women race the same course as the men. Women cover the same terrain under the same conditions, and sometimes cover it faster than the men. For these athletes, Ironman is empowering; Ironman provides a neutral playing field for male and female competitors alike, a feat only feasible due to the hard work and ceaseless commitment of women who demanded the right to play and do so in a climate that would not allow it.

Respect is an important issue for NY, an accomplished sixty-three-year-old female athlete. She commented,

Women are often not given their due for what they do, and I think in athletics there's the clock, and so there are certain things that demarcate what you do, and it does improve your self-image, and I think in triathlon, especially if you're older. A lot of older people don't get any credit for doing what they do because they're older, but I think in triathlon you do, because younger people want to be like you when they're your age—they want to participate—so they give you the respect that you may not get in any other, in a lot of other fields.

Given the unique inception of the Ironman triathlon and the historical inclusion of women in the race, this particular athlete is able to capture the climate of Ironman racing in her statement.

To summarize the qualitative findings on body type, 30% of Ironman athletes believe there is an Ironman body type while 47% believe there is not an Ironman body type. Forty-seven percent of athletes interviewed believe that the Ironman body type differs from the social ideal for female beauty while 23% believe it does not. Ironman bodies were described as *mentally tough, muscular/toned, fit, strong, lean, healthy, skinny, thin, balanced*. Ironman athletes described the social conception of ideal beauty as *skinny, fit, toned, supermodel/Barbie, lean. Fit, skinny,* and *lean* were words used both to describe Ironman body types and the social aesthetic. While 70% of athletes interviewed believed that women were respected in the racing realm and none believed they were not, Ironman athletes still show signs of adhering to a social aesthetic when four of the seven words used to describe Ironman bodies are the same words Ironman athletes use to describe a social aesthetic.

Males and females both fall prey to a cultural mandate for thinness, and thus, when exercise is used to achieve a certain appearance—to make the body look a certain way to others—then the body is an object, and Ironman racing becomes a means to an end (a way of justifying an exercise addiction or a way of obtaining a socially pleasing body). If, however, exercise is used to make it possible for the body to do certain things, like completing an Ironman, then the body is an agent, and Ironman is not just a means to an end, but rather the end itself. The distinction between subject and object is not so overt; there are moments when Ironman athletes are agentic and subjects of their own control, and there are moments when they are objects, acting in pursuit of a social aesthetic. Ironman athletes report this very tension in their simultaneously distinct yet repetitive language describing Ironman body types and a cultural aesthetic. While some words are different, others are the same, highlighting the tension and overlap between the potential moments where Ironman athletes are empowered and disempowered by their athletic pursuits.

Postmodern feminist theory offers an explanation for this tension, as female Ironman athletes are discursive subjects who come into being through their very interaction both in and outside of the Ironman racing realm. According to Bordo (1993), there is no body prior to its marking; both literally and figuratively, bodies become marked as Ironman athletes through the numbering ritual before each race. Officials write with permanent marker on athletes' arms and legs for the purpose of identifying competitors throughout the race. According to Hilliard (1988), athletes enter into the subculture of triathlon through the body-marking process itself. Both while marked and unmarked, however, female Ironman athletes are always both females and athletes, influenced by a social aesthetic and a desire to race fast. Their overlap in word choice highlights this possible attempt for female Ironman athletes to bring their participation in Ironman into alignment with a social norm of aesthetically pleasing bodies, in the historical legacy of sport as a masculine domain. The repetition of adjectives used to describe cultural ideals of beauty and Ironman bodies potentially points to the place where Ironman can be used as a means to an end of obtaining the aesthetically pleasing body. Thus female Ironman athletes articulate the complexity of Ironman as empowering and Ironman as disempowering.

SATAQ-3R scores confirmed that Ironman athletes are highly cognizant of their bodies, and themes that emerged from interview data highlight the "extreme" nature of Ironman training and racing. Thus, according to Duncan (1994), Ironman athletes are disempowered by their athletic pursuits as they "continually monitor their bodies for imperfections" and "exercising to extremes" (p. 54). However, there is another argument to be made for the Ironman athlete.

The very fact that women *can* change their bodies in the attempt to mimic a social aesthetic (which changes over time and is different in different locales) simultaneously destabilizes the naturalized female body and enables women to create a new definition of femininity and beauty, specifically because, as Moore (1997) wrote, "malleable flesh [is] abstractly molded by power" (p. 5). Flesh can be molded. According to Grosz (1994), individuals develop identity "from the outside in." In other words, through social inscriptions on the body, or punishment and reward, according to Butler (1990, 1993, 1997), individuals enact a rigid and coherent gendered identity as prescripted and policed by society (power). Ironman athletes in this study attempted to align their Ironman identity within a rigid social aesthetic and cohere their, at times, dichotomous identities (as females in a male bastion of sport) by using the same words to describe Ironman bodies and a cultural notion of beauty. They are taking their identity from the "outside" and from different systems of power, both in and outside of the Ironman racing realm, and making their identity on the "inside" cohere.

Data collected in this study support the finding from DiGioacchino et al. (2002b) that female and male triathletes are very concerned about their body. DiGioacchino et al. found 29% of males and 49% of females reported being "sometimes, or always, terrified about being overweight." Twenty-one percent of males and 47% of females were "sometimes, or always, preoccupied with the desire to be thinner." Twenty-eight percent of males and 43% of females were "sometimes, or always, preoccupied with the thought of having fat on their body" (p. 217). Further research is necessary to deduce whether this fear is motivated by a desire to race faster or a desire to appear aesthetically pleasing. In either case data in this study confirm DiGioacchino et al.'s findings that triathletes are highly concerned with their appearance.

Table 9

Comparison of SATAQ-3R Results with College Norms and Eating Disorder Patients

	Current Project (n = 40: 27 M, 13 F)		College Norms (n = 380)		Eating Disorder Patients (n = 326)	
	Mean	*SD*	Mean	*SD*	Mean	*SD*
Total SATAQ Scores						
Males	116.1	18.6	NA	NA	NA	NA
Females	108.2	20.8**	NA	NA	NA	NA
Information						
Males	39.2	5.8	NA	NA	NA	NA
Females	37.2	8.6	31.2 *	10.1	29.9 *	9.7
Pressures						
Males	30.2	6.1	NA	NA	NA	NA
Females	26.7	7.0	22.5 *	8.3	26.4	7.7
Internalization–General						
Males	36.3	8.5	NA	NA	NA	NA
Females	35.5	9.1	28.7 *	9.8	34.7	9.2
Internalization–Athlete						
Males	20.5	4.7**	NA	NA	NA	NA
Females	18.1	4.7	16.2 *	4.9	18.1	4.5

*p = <.05

**significant kurtosis

† Source: "The Sociocultural Attitudes Towards Appearance Scale-3" by Thompson, van den Berg, Roehrig, Guarda, & Heinberg, 2004, *International Journal of Eating Disorders, 35*, pp. 299

†† Source: "The Sociocultural Attitudes Towards Appearance Questionnaire (SATAQ-3): Reliability and normative comparisons of eating disorder patients" by R. Calogero, W. Davis and J. Thompson, 2004, *Body Image, 1*, p. 196.

Female and male Ironman athletes in the sample did not score significantly differently from one another on the SATAQ-3R. The female total SATAQ-3R score demonstrated significant kurtosis and thus must be interpreted somewhat cautiously. Males scored higher than female Ironman athletes in all four subcategories. Female Ironman athletes scored significantly higher than college females on the SATAQ-3R in all subcategories of the SATAQ-3R: information, pressures, internalization–general, internalization–athlete. Female Ironman athletes scored significantly higher than eating-disorder patients in the subcategory Information. Thus, I can conclude, based on my quantitative data, that Ironman athletes, at least females, are significantly influenced by social attitudes toward appearance.

Given that college norms are the "healthy" baseline data, Ironman athletes score higher than females with eating disorders on the SATAQ-3R. In answering question number four—to what extent are male and female Ironman athletes influenced by social attitudes toward gender-appropriate appearance on the SATAQ?—I can conclude based on my quantitative data that Ironman athletes, at least females, are in fact significantly influenced by social attitudes toward appearance.

Triangulation of Demographic Data SATAQ-3R and EDQ

To answer the fifth research question—how do athletes' attitudes toward appearance affect their propensity for exercise addiction?—demographic data, subscales from the SATAQ-3R, and subscales from the EDQ were triangulated. Spearman Rho correlations and p values were calculated for the total EDQ scores and subscales and plotted against total SATAQ-3R total scores and subscales. Data were separated out for gender.

Females who exercise for weight reasons score significantly higher on the SATAQ-3R total scale and internalization–general and internalization–athlete subscales. These women accept messages regarding unrealistic ideals for attractiveness, and they endorse and accept the relatively new athletic and "toned" body ideal. Females who score higher on the insight into problem subscale of the EDQ also score higher on the SATAQ subscales of pressure (feel pressure from exposure to media and messages to modify appearance) and internalization–general. Thus women who score higher on the insight into problems scale are much more concerned about their weight and tend to score higher on the body-image scale.

Males who exercise for positive-reward values are more likely to score higher for total SATAQ-3R, internalization–general, pressures (wherein one feels pressure from exposure to media and messages to modify one's appearance). For total EDQ and internalization–general, males who scored higher on the EDQ were more likely to accept messages portraying unrealistic ideals for attractiveness and strive toward these ideals. In summary, these findings support the conclusion that the higher Ironman athletes score on the SATAQ-3R, the more athletes strive to obtain specified ideals of beauty/athleticism through exercise.

While no other study has been done investigating social attitudes toward appearance and exercise dependence, Blaydon and Lindner (2002) studied the correlation between eating attitudes and exercise dependence in triathletes. They found that 12.3% of tested triathletes had Eating Attitudes Test (EAT) scores indicative of an eating disorder, 30.4% tested to have pathological levels of exercise dependence and 21.6% had elevated EAT *and* EDQ scores. A total of 64.3% of researched triathletes tested to have positive scores for one of the following three dependence patterns: an eating disorder, an exercise dependence, or an eating disorder *and* an exercise dependence. Thus, according to Blaydon and Lindner's findings, triathletes in the 2002 study have a higher incidence of exercise dependence without an associated eating disorder. However, the fact that over half of the test population scored in the pathological range in one of the dependence patterns under investigation is a startling finding and one supported by this research project. My results showed that 55% of Ironman triathletes scored above the cutoff for exercise dependence and are highly influenced by a social aesthetic. In fact, this research adds to Blaydon and Linder's contentions, both because it further narrows the population to Ironman distance triathletes and because data from this project suggest a positively correlated relationship between internalized attitudes toward appearance and exercise dependence. It is important to note that withdrawal, a central concept of exercise dependence, was not significantly associated with the SATAQ-3R findings.

Table 10 and Table 11 present the correlations between the SATAQ and the EDQ for females and males respectively.

Table 10

Spearman Rho Correlations and p-Values for Females on the Total SATAQ and EDQ Scales and Subscales.

	Total SATAQ	Information	Pressures	Internalization– general	Internalization– athlete
Total EDQ	.43(.14)	.13(.67)	.19(.52)	.51(.07)	.31(.30)
Interference	.29(.33)	.29(.33)	.12(.70)	.05(.86)	.09(.76)
Positive reward	.40(.18)	.15(.62)	.28(.35)	.46(.11)	.22(.47)
Withdrawal	.28(.35)	.36(.23)	.22(.47)	.44(.14)	.04(.90)
Exercise—weight	.56(.045)*	.20(.52)	.25(.41)	.71(.01)*	.59(.04)*
Insight	.70(.01)*	.48(.10)	.57(.04)*	.66(.01)*	.34(.26)
Exercise—social	-.20(.52)	-.26(.39)	.20(.51)	-.14(.66)	-.07(.83)
Exercise—health	-.06(.85)	-.36(.23)	-.01(.97)	.06(.85)	.36(.22)
Stereotyped behavior	-.007(.98)	-.31(.32)	-.33(.27)	.18(.55)	.19(.54)

*indicates significant correlation ($p < .05$)

In summary these findings support the conclusion that the higher Ironman athletes score on the SATAQ-3R, the more athletes strive to obtain specified ideals of beauty/athleticism through exercise. Specifically, males who demonstrated high levels of exercise for positive reward values on the EDQ were more likely to score higher on the SATAQ-3R subcategories: internalization–general and pressure. Females who exercise for weight reasons scored significantly higher on the SATAQ-3R total scale and internalization–general and internalization–athlete subscales. Females who scored higher on the insight into problem subscale of the EDQ also scored higher on the SATAQ-3R subscales of pressure and internalization–general.

Table 11

Spearman Rho Correlations and p-Values for Males on the Total SATAQ and EDQ
Scales and Subscales.

	Total SATAQ	Information	Pressures	Internalization–general	Internalization–athlete
Total EDQ	.27(.17)	.02(.91)	.08(.70)	.41(.04)*	.18(.37)
Interference	-.20(.32)	-.06(.76)	-.27(.17)	-.07(.72)	-.07(.74)
Positive reward	.49(.01)*	.14(.48)	.39(.046)*	.47(.01)*	.03(.90)
Withdrawal	.23(.25)	.11(.58)	-.02(.93)	.27(.17)	.03(.89)
Exercise—weight	.11(.58)	-.36(.07)	.15(.47)	.23(.24)	.03(.89)
Insight	.21(.30)	.08(.69)	.13(.51)	.33(.10)	.35(.08)
Exercise—social	.29(.14)	.37(.06)	-.04(.83)	.30(.13)	.15(.47)
Exercise—health	.08(.68)	-.14(.49)	.05(.82)	.08(.70)	.19(.36)
Stereotyped behavior	.22(.27)	-.20(.33)	.17(.41)	.34(.08)	.12(.57)

*indicates significant correlation ($p < .05$)

Hausenblas and Downs (2002b) noted "men reported more exercise dependence symptoms than women." My quantitative data corroborates Hausenblas and Downs' findings that males report more exercise addiction than females. Males in this study scored higher on the SATAQ-3R than females, and a higher percentage of males scored in the pathological range on the EDQ than females. Most of my qualitative data came from females, while a large percentage of my quantitative came from males. The triathlon community is still predominantly male, and because an e-mail dissemination was used to solicit survey participants, a larger sampling of men were targeted and subsequently contributed to my findings. When I administered interviews, I was able target female athletes.

Caution must be used in triangulating the findings in the quantitative and qualitative data due to the small sample size as well as the demographic discrepancy between the two samples. While my quantitative data is more supportive of the concept of exercise addiction and its relation to the sociocultural ideals of beauty than my qualitative data, this is perhaps due to the short duration of the interviews as well as the self-selection bias for those who agreed to be interviewed, ultimately limiting the extent to which people were willing to acknowledge that they might have problems. In contrast, the advertisement used to recruit participants for online survey participation may have biased participation to those particularly willing to acknowledge problems. Even though all data were collected from Ironmen, caution must be used in triangulating the findings, because it is possible that the two-phase data collection sampled two different subpopulations of Ironman athletes.

Reflections—what does it all mean?

Reading over the criteria for what constitutes exercise dependence, I found myself displaying strong signs of exercise dependence, and wondered how many other triathletes shared my fate by the mere fact that they trained for and raced in an Ironman competition. My question is: do exercise addicts flock to triathlon to justify their addiction, or does triathlon breed exercise addiction by the nature of the competition and the demands of the training? While my research did not attempt to disentangle this cause-and-effect relationship, it did provide a more complete and cohesive picture of the triathlon community. Who is an Ironman triathlete? What does he/she think about gender, about his/her body, about his/her training, and about his/her motivations and identity as a triathlete? Using a combination of qualitative and quantitative data, I sought to paint a picture of the triathlon subculture, complete with commonalities and aberrations—individuals who race to eat, who race to run from the bottle, who race to find purpose, and who race for fun, exhilaration, and the sheer challenge of it all. This is the Ironman athlete I found; this is the Ironman athlete I embody, I coach, and I listen to and learn from.

While Ironman athletes take pride in their accomplishments ("extreme" endeavors), they also recognize the unique mentality Ironman requires/attracts and freely admit that Ironman has the potential to become "obsessive." Quantitative findings support qualitative interview data as both male and female Ironman athletes demonstrated higher levels of exercise dependence than Zmijewski and Howard's (2003) control population. Findings also revealed that levels of exercise dependence for both male and female Ironman athletes are influenced by the extent to which social attitudes toward appearance are internalized. The more Ironman athletes internalize a cultural aesthetic of beauty, the more they strive to obtain that aesthetic through exercise (in this case Ironman training). Thus research suggests that the prevalence of exercise dependence among Ironman athletes is dictated by the individual's purpose for Ironman participation. If Ironman participation is in pursuit of a social aesthetic, then exercise-dependence patterns are more likely to exist. If, however, Ironman participation is motivated by reasons other than an internalization and drive to obtain a social aesthetic, the exercise-dependence patterns will not be demonstrated, despite the rigorous training regime necessary to complete an Ironman triathlon. This research concludes that not all Ironman athletes are exercise dependent and yet based on their commitment and sheer volume spent training, their participation alone marks them as addicts, according to current concepts concerning exercise addiction. Also, not all female Ironman athletes are empowered individuals; some, in fact, are highly influenced by a social aesthetic and do demonstrate exercise dependence patterns for the purpose of weight control.

By examining both the bodies and the systems that shape those bodies, this work contributes to the field of postmodern feminist inquiry, sport studies, and psychology through the critical investigation into exercise addiction and Ironman athletes. My research concludes that while Ironman has the potential to become obsessive, not all Ironman athletes are addicts, and while Ironman has the potential to be empowering, not all who race Ironman are, in fact, empowered.

Chapter 4: Physiology: Overtraining

The previous three chapters have outlined an academic account of exercise addiction in endurance athletes. What follows is an integration of this research into an accessible application of this knowledge so that coaches, mental health practitioners, and the self-coached or inquisitive athlete can benefit from this new information. As a coach or a self-coached athlete, it is a challenging balance to push just beyond limits and then to build in recovery time. This method allows the body to reap the benefits of exertion. This is how an athlete gets stronger. If athletes are not overloaded and then rested, they do not improve; when pushed too much without proper rest, they get injured, sick, or burned out. This challenge is a struggle for every coach. Exercise-dependent athletes want to train hard every single day, which is simply not healthy and not physiologically sound. This also doesn't produce the optimal training load and subsequent adaptation.

Overtraining syndrome is a much-contested issue in the field of exercise physiology, much like exercise addiction in the psychological realm. Overtraining refers to the experience of "staleness" on the part of an athlete. When athletes are not performing at their optimal level, coaches and physiologists look at every component of an athlete's training, which may include all of the following:

Psychological: How is their mood state? Are they energized, depressed, tired, or anxious?

Biochemical: What is their red blood cell count? Are they anemic? What is their white blood cell count? Are they fighting an infection?

Hormonal: What is their cortisol level? Are they stressed?

Even the autonomic nervous system can sometimes be monitored for signs of overtraining. More specific accounts in this area of research are described below.

Physiologists Halson and Jeukendrup (2004) reviewed the literature in the field of exercise physiology and concluded, "The general lack of research in the area in combination with very few well-controlled investigations means that it is very difficult to gain insight into the incidence, markers, and possible causes of overtraining" (p. 968). And yet overtraining exists; "20–60% of athletes experience the negative effects of overtraining at least once during their career" (Urhausen and Kindermann 2002, p. 819). As such, it is important that coaches are familiar with the signs and symptoms as well as some theories contributing to overtraining to avoid these occurrences in their athletes.

Urhausen and Kindermann (2002) assessed the myriad of ways in which overtraining syndrome has been evaluated. Every component of the human body has been examined for signs and possible explanations of evidence of overtraining. Researchers studied heart rate, hormone levels, psychological changes, and enzymatic metabolic markers in the blood. To date, sport-specific performance, ergometric performance, neuromuscular excitability, mood profiles, subjective complaints, Borg scale, heart rate, respiratory exchange ratio, lactate, conductive keratoplasty and urea, testosterone, cortisol, adrenocorticotropic hormone, and finally catecholamines have been investigated in overtraining-syndrome research. Fourteen different methods were used to measure overtraining, and none was conclusive.

While a lack of conclusive research exists, the prevalence of the symptomology is real. According to Lehmann et al. (1997), overtraining remains a somewhat common although much misunderstood phenomenon in sport. The "unexplained underperformance" is one diagnosis adopted among physiologists, coaches, and athletes alike. Looking to exercise addiction could be one possible explanation for underperformance.

Detecting exercise dependence patterns is the first step in producing healthy and successful athletes. Noting when athletes refuse to rest, become agitated during periods of taper, or prioritize training over family, work, and social obligations are warning signs that exercise dependence may be present. It is incumbent upon the coach to recognize these warning signs and employ a team approach by calling on the help of a mental health practitioner. The coach is often the first line of defense here, as he/ she can monitor an athlete's progress and the attitude with which the athlete approaches his/her training. While exercise dependence is still not a DSM-diagnosed illness, mental-health practitioners will be better able to help their clients when they are able to identify and understand both the signs and symptoms of exercise dependence patterns.

And while "treatment" is yet unexamined, simply not training will produce marked withdrawal symptoms. Mental-health practitioners, coaches, and athletes can become aware of these behavior patterns and engage in open dialogue about their exercise dependence. Now that SATAQ-3R scores have been correlated with EDQ scores and subset patterns, perhaps the road to treatment lies in disentangling one's quest for a thin social aesthetic with their exercise regime.

From Theory to Practice

When athletes become overtrained, they often notice a decrease in their performance, a mood disturbance, a shift in their appetite resulting in a potential change in their body composition, an alternation in their sleep habits, and an alteration in their overall affect. Athletes who exhibit signs of exercise addiction are particularly prone to suffering from overtraining, as they are unable to take rest days. Their performance suffers as they are not able to disentangle the cause of the issue from the result. In other words, performance suffers because of inadequate recovery, and yet athletes, instead of resting, increase their training volume under the false premise that their declines in performance are due to inadequate training. This is, in fact, the opposite of what they need; increasing training volume and intensity serves to exacerbate the problem, not rectify it. The longer athletes continue along their path of overtraining, the further they dig themselves into a hole, making recovery time longer.

As a coach and as a member of the endurance community, I have heard far too many stories of athletes whose first event was their fastest. With more and more training, their race times increased, not decreased.

They spend increasingly more hours training and attempt to ramp up the intensity (although they are often unable to) only to post slower and slower race results. This is a very clear sign of overtraining, and while the rationale for training more to rectify slower times seems reasonable, it is antithetical to what the athlete actually needs for faster times. Rest is what athletes need to pull themselves out of an underrecovery spiral which is severely affecting not only their athletic results, but also their overall health. And yet rest is very challenging, if not virtually impossible for exercise addicts, for rest deprives them of their addictive substance (exercise).

So, how do we apply all of this research to training? With the advent of heart rate monitors, power meters, and data analysis software, athletes and coaches are now able to quantify and track training stress and monitor recovery. Coaches and athletes can use the available technology to prevent overtraining from occurring using the following methods.

Profile of Mood State

Coaches, mental health practitioners, and self-coached athletes can utilize the Profile of Mood States to track levels of specific emotions throughout a training cycle. Monitoring mental health, or at least intensities of particular emotions, which the POMS can do, serves to document trends in an athlete's mood and can offer insight into correlations between moods, reactions to particular workouts, and overall emotional health throughout the course of a training block. It can quantify a qualitative trend a coach or athlete may detect, and it can serve as a valuable addition to any training log. After all, an athlete's emotional health is intricately tied with his/her physical health, and his/her sporting performance.

The Profile of Mood State (POMS) generally begins with a question such as, "Fill in one space under the answer that best describes how you have been feeling in the past hour." The five-point scale is given as follows: not at all (1), a little (2), moderately (3), quite a bit (4), extremely (5).

- Friendly
- Tense
- Angry
- Worn Out
- Unhappy
- Clear-headed
- Lively
- Confused
- Sorry for things done
- Shaky
- Listless
- Peeved
- Considerate
- Sad
- Active
- On edge
- Grouchy
- Blue
- Energetic
- Panicky
- Hopeless
-
-

- Relaxed
- Unworthy
- Spiteful
- Sympathetic
- Uneasy
- Restless
- Unable to concentrate
- Fatigued
- Helpful
- Annoyed
- Discouraged
- Resentful
- Nervous
- Lonely
- Miserable
- Muddled
- Cheerful
- Bitter
- Exhausted
- Anxious
- Ready to fight
-
-

- Good-natured
- Gloomy
- Desperate
- Sluggish
- Rebellious
- Helpless
- Weary
- Bewildered
- Alert
- Deceived
- Furious
- Efficacious
- Trusting
- Full of pep
- Bad-tempered
- Worthless
- Forgetful
- Carefree
- Terrified
- Guilty
- Vigorous
- Uncertain about things
- Bushed

The following short form is another alternative to administering the POMS. The same five-point scale is given as follows: not at all (1), a little, moderately (2), quite a bit (3), extremely (4).

- tense
- depressed
- angry
- vigorous
- fatigued
- confused

Scoring POMS: Add up your total score and use it as a baseline for subsequent inventories. Watch trends both in cumulative score and individual mood states and include POMS scores in training logs in order to monitor mental and emotional health.

Training Logs

Athletes do not exist in a vacuum. They are influenced by the world around them, their training, and their progression as athletes. This pursuit cannot be isolated to only their training sessions proper. Instead, their sleep, their hydration, their nutrition, their energy levels, their stress levels, their psychological health, their rate of recovery, all affect their progress as athletes. Training logs help to monitor the multifaceted aspects of an athlete beyond their physical training. Training logs also help to establish patterns and trends in athletes that cannot always be discerned in the present moment. Looking back over an athlete's training log history, a coach or a self-coached athlete may be able to detect commonalities that elicit insight into the present moment. Why is an athlete not responding properly to training? Answers to this question and other questions will become evident once the training log is studied. Answers to these questions may not be possible to uncover with only the presenting facts of the day or week.

Athletes should keep training logs that include the following information:
1) Sleep—hours and quality
2) Body weight and body composition—to be measured weekly at the same time of day
3) Workout specifics—discipline, volume, intensity
4) Workout comments—how the workout was executed, how it felt, what was consumed throughout the workout: amount of fluid, kcal, and electrolytes
5) Hydration—how much fluid was consumed throughout the day
6) Caffeine level—how much caffeine was ingested
7) Nutrition—total kcal or percentage of macronutrients consumed
8) Stress level—work, family, and social stresses
9) Overall mental and physical health—note any illness or injury

Athletes should keep detailed accounts not only of their workouts, but also what happens throughout their day apart from their workouts. The athlete is an amalgamation of his/her entire experience; how he/she performs in a training session may very well have to do with what happened outside of the training session. Was his/her nutrition off? Did he/she get enough sleep? Is he/she stressed out because of something else in life? Merely recording mile times and heart rates is not sufficient to optimize sporting performance, because more than an athlete's workout determines athletic progress. It is the combination of his/her workout and everything else throughout a twenty-four-hour day.

There are many options when it comes to monitoring training and daily logs. A simple journal will suffice, or there are a host of online resources that can serve as a storage and scrutiny sy4stem3 allowing for observation of trends through graphic functions.

Heart Rate

By monitoring resting heart rate, coaches and athletes can watch heart rate trends. A rising resting heart rate can indicate that an athlete is either not fully recovered from the previous training stress or is likely coming down with a cold or other viral illnesses. If resting heart rate is elevated, it is advised that athletes should skip their planned workout, or make it a recovery day, performing only very light exercise for less than sixty minutes. Monitoring resting heart rate over the course of a training cycle will provide valuable information on how the athlete is progressing in terms of fitness (one can expect resting heart rate to decrease with training). It can also measure how well athletes are responding to and recovering from increased training volume and intensity.

Monitoring heart rate while training can also be a valuable tool to identify overtraining. If heart rate is elevated above normal levels during activity or specific intervals, it is possible that the athlete is not fully recovered and not ready for subsequent training. Again, an off day or recovery day is advised. It is also advisable to watch for potential signs of dehydration, as an elevated heart rate during training can be a sign of dehydration as well.

Power

With the increased use of power meters, athletes are better able to quantify the work they perform during their training. Power meters accurately measure workload in a specified training session and monitor cumulative workload throughout an entire block of training. They also can help indicate when an athlete is not fully rested and not able to perform up to his/her potential. During training using power meters, if an athlete is unable to reach his/her prescribed ranges, he/she might need additional rest and recovery. Athletes should not continue their workout if their power drops below 10% of their prescribed range.

Data analysis software can help a coach monitor overload and recovery throughout an athlete's week, month, and year to ensure there is a proper systematic build in terms of intensity and volume, and adequate recovery between workout blocks. By mapping total stress scores alongside intensity factors, coaches and athletes can literally quantify the stress they are undergoing throughout their training cycles. Software such as TrainingPeaks and PowerAgent offer in-depth graphing functions to help monitor overload and recovery.

Preventing Overtraining

I have found the singular best way to prevent overtraining is to hire a coach. It is invaluable to have an objective opinion. Hiring an informed professional to design a physiologically sound training plan builds in a prevention plan to avoid overtraining. I have often quipped that a coach "saves me from myself," and this is all too true. Ironically, I am a coach, but I am a horrible self-coach. I know this about myself, so I utilize the expertise of other coaches who can structure a sound training plan and offer advice when needed.

The problem many athletes face when executing a training plan is just that: the rigid adherence to executing a training plan. If the ultimate goal is to go faster on race day, that may very well mean skipping a workout when resting heart rate is elevated or the beginnings of an injury are presenting themselves. Athletes who are prone to exhibit signs of exercise addiction have a very hard time making this decision to skip a day for overall health and wellness and optimal success. There is no forest for the trees, there are only trees—and a coach can help an athlete refocus on the forest.

For exercise addicts, training becomes an integral part of their identity. What began as a healthy coping strategy evolved into an added stress and an additional obligation. What once was an enjoyable activity now rules one's life to unhealthy extremes. Coaches and mental health practitioners can help athletes develop additional coping strategies and a multifaceted sense of self. Exercise is not the singular attribute of an individual, nor is it his/her only coping skill. I discuss this more in the next chapter.

How to avoid overtraining:

1. Have a training plan with systematic and progressive overload—a three-week build and one-week recovery is standard practice. See table 12 below as a sample training plan that incorporates progressive build and adequate recovery.

Table 12

Wk of:	Monday	Tuesday	Wednesday	Thursday	Friday	Saturday	Sunday	Totals
8-Jun	Strength training 30 min	1 hr run with 30 min tempo at 155-158 heart rate	Strength training 30 min	off	90 min hike or bike,	Run 90 minutes trail	Run 60 minutes trail	5:30 total
15-Jun	Strength training 30 min	1 hr run with 40 min tempo at 155-158 heart rate	Strength training 30 min	off	90 min hike or bike,	Run 2 hrs trail	Run 90 minutes trail	6:30 total
22-Jun	Strength training 30 min	1 hr run with 45 min tempo at 155-158 heart rate	Strength training 30 min	off	45 min run	60 min run	off	7:00 total
29-Jun	Strength training 30 min	45 min run	Strength training 30 min	1hr	90 min hike or bike,	Run 1:30 hrs trail	swim	4:15 total

Allow ample recovery between efforts, between blocks of training, and between goal events.

2. Monitor progress and recovery through daily logs, paying particular attention to:
    - progress in training—increases in speed and power, decreases in heart rate
    - race results
    - nutrition, hydration, electrolyte replacement
    - appetite
    - body composition
    - sleep—amount and quality
    - resting heart rate
    - energy levels
    - attitudes—POMS
    - daily stress—work, family, friends
    - illness and injury
    - utilize training tools such as heart rate and power meters

3. Education. When athletes understand the importance of recovery in their training program, they are more likely to follow the program as written. Read about exercise physiology and how the body responds to overload. Understand that the body gets stronger and adapts to stress only in the recovery and rest phases. Too much overload leads to injury and illness and thus negatively affects performance. Athletes need to be aware of all of the contributing factors when it comes to their training, including the importance of sleep, proper nutrition, minimizing stress, and recognizing early signs of overtraining or inadequate recovery. The more educated athletes are about the process of training, the better equipped they are to avoid the potentials of overtraining. They understand the ramifications of their actions, namely negative performance, and can become their own best advocates

when it comes to training healthy and racing strong. Athletes are the first line of defense when it comes to avoiding overtraining. Coaches and mental health practitioners can be scrupulous about the data collection and monitoring of overload and recovery, but, arguably, no one knows his/her body better than the athlete himself/herself. Education can provide the tools to know what to look for in early detection of problematic patterns and thus enable athletes to avoid the slippery slope of overtraining.

Athletes, whether self-coached or working with a coach, should learn about exercise addiction and overtraining; it is important information. Even while someone else may be prescribing workouts, an athlete can still suffer from an exercise addiction and can still fall prey to overtraining. Being a coached athlete does not let an athlete off the hook from evaluating his/her own levels of addiction and dependence. In fact, taking a closer look at one's relationship with exercise may very well help one's coach provide the best training possible, resulting in an athlete's race day successes. While a coach can help prescribe daily workouts, the attitude with which athletes approach their training and their ability to rest and recover still comes down to them, and their own levels of addiction or dependence.

Beyond performance, taking a close and hard look at one's own potential dependence and/or addiction to exercise can help pull an athlete out of a detrimental pattern which invariably leads to overtraining and a compromised quality of life. Athletes are looking to race fast. They are also seeking health and balance; the two are not mutually exclusive. In fact, learning to rest, recover, and have a healthy approach to training and exercise will lead to faster race-day results. An overtrained athlete is not a fast athlete. An exercise addict is almost always overtrained or underrecovered because he/she does not know how to rest. In the next chapter, I offer some tools as to how to approach rest and recovery, be it a planned day off or an unplanned injury.

Chapter 5: Survival Skills for an Off Day

Okay, so now the athlete knows what exercise addiction is, knows how to test for his/her own levels, and can monitor training stress with gadgets and gizmos to avoid overtraining. So what? What are athletes to do with all of this newfound knowledge? In this chapter I offer tips for off days and skills for surviving a missed workout. It's not easy—trust me, I know—but it happens from time to time. The athlete spikes a fever, or his/her kid does, the boss calls with an unrealistic deadline, and the two-hour training plan that was squeezed into the day really needs to be devoted to something else now. How does one plan for the eventuality of the unknown?

I spent a whole lot of time talking about addiction and how athletes who are addicted can't make reasonable decisions when it comes to their workouts, but the bottom line is that despite the level of addiction, an athlete sometimes has to take a day off. What follows are some techniques and advice on how to approach this "blessing in disguise" without it throwing the athlete for a loop. Athletes have options when eventualities beyond their control shake their perfectly laid plans. Options include getting angry, resentful, mean, sad, depressed, pissed off at the world—or rolling with it.

Some would take the above scenarios as a blessing—a day off, an excuse not to train—but not exercise addicts. No, exercise addicts are so wed to their training that they don't know what to do with themselves when they cannot train. Addicts can become irritable, anxious, and/or depressed on scheduled off days. Their sense of self is so tied to their ability to exercise that without that outlet they are literally lost. My recommendation is to create other outlets, other facets of self. What else brings happiness? Sure, exercise is a wonderful outlet—when balanced. But what else brings a smile? Gardening? Spending time with friends or loved ones? Cooking? Reading? Watching a movie? Developing other talents and hobbies can help establish balance that exercise addicts lack.

Balance simply doesn't make sense to the exercise addict. He/she wants more and more and *needs* to work out longer and longer in order to get his/her fix. This is not balance; this is the "tolerance" effect of an addiction—the need to increase the stimulant in order to reach the same desired effects. In this case, the stimulant is exercise, and the desired effects may be a runner's high, a sense of accomplishment, and a desire to burn calories. There are a number of desired effects associated with exercise. As my research concludes, the more athletes train to make their body look a certain way, the higher the incidence of exercise addiction. So, if the desired effect of exercise is to lose weight or shape the body in a particular way, the likelihood of exercise addiction is relatively high.

The counterargument here is that to be highly successful at anything, it takes dedication and singular focus as well as a lean build. While I agree to a certain extent, even pros take days off, and even pros can under-nourish and suffer from the detrimental effects of depleting their body's necessary nutrients. Professional athletes realize the need to know how to rest, relax, and develop other aspects of their identity. Because rest and recovery are so crucial to their success, they comprehend the signifi-cance of staying as stress free as possible. Increasing undue stress can lead to both injury and illness due to increased levels of cortisol, a catabolic hormone, in the body. Thus, reducing stress enhances recovery by limiting the elevation of cortisol.

Injury/Illness

Exercise addicts are more prone to suffer from injury and illness because they don't rest and recover adequately. As mentioned earlier in the text, the first incidents of exercise addiction were recorded by ortho-pedists who were seeing runners who presented like drug addicts looking for the next high. They needed their fix (running) and they were unable to get it due to an overuse injury. Progressive build and adequate recovery will enable the body to grow stronger through training. Without this systematized approach, an athlete is much more susceptible to injury. When the body is depleted through too much overload and inadequate recovery, the immune system becomes depressed and the incidence for illness is higher.

So the athlete suffers from illness or injury; he/she knows he/she overdid it and vows to take more rest days in the future. Now what? What is the athlete to do right now to help get through to the other side of this injury or illness? As a certified athletic trainer, I have seen many athletes suffer from injury and illness. Here are some psychological tools to help recovery.

Believe it or not, athletes go through a grieving process when they become injured. Most athletes go through all five stages of grief:

1. Denial—Training through the injury, pretending it doesn't exist.
2. Anger—The athlete becomes mad that the injury or illness happened at this inopportune time (as if there is ever an opportune time for injury or illness).
3. Bargaining—The athlete vows to change his/her behaviors, to take more rest days in the future, to not overdo it next time.
4. Depression—The athlete becomes withdrawn and wallows in self-pity.
5. Acceptance—The athlete no longer resists the present moment, but instead accept it as it is. This is when the healing can begin.

It is helpful for the athlete to dialogue with someone about his/her feelings in order to facilitate moving through all five stages and arriving at acceptance. Talking to a coach, a mentor, running buddies, or a doctor is helpful. Athletes need to acknowledge feelings and verbalize grief in order to move through the five stages of emotion. Denying feelings does not help healing. It only keeps the athlete stuck in stage one.

While the present moment feels like forever, an athlete needs to remember that it is not. He/she needs to know that even though he/she may not be able to train today, he/she will, most likely, be able to train again in the future. Many athletes dramatize the present moment into the eternal; this is not helpful.

What is helpful is hearing about another person's full recovery from injury. One highly successful athlete I coach suffered a terrible crash on her bike. She was poised to place in all of her upcoming races, and yet she was scheduled for surgery to have a plate put in her shattered arm. The season we had spent so long preparing for came and went. But this athlete worked hard in her rehab, ran "miles" in the deep end of the pool, pedaled on her trainer, and returned to racing the following season to clinch her Kona slot. The injury was devastating at first, but once we were able to refocus on the following year, she was able to put her injury in perspective, grieve the loss of one season, and look ahead to the following year. The present moment, while painful physically and emotionally, did not last forever. Through a shift in attention from the immediacy of what was lost to the potential for all that could be gained in another year's time, she was able to overcome her injury, fully heal, and return to competition as strong, if not stronger, than she was before her crash.

Talking to other athletes who have also suffered from an injury and have returned to activity can be both comforting and inspirational. It can remind the athlete that others have suffered from injuries; it can help to reiterate that the present moment is not forever, and it can keep the athlete connected to community while not participating in the target sport.

It is also helpful to be well informed about the recovery process. Speaking to a physician or physical therapist can be instrumental in the recovery process. Gaining as much information as possible enables the athlete to approach the injury or illness from a logical and educated standpoint instead of an emotional one.

Emotions are not all negative, though. An athlete can stay positive and facilitate the healing process. The injury happened; one's response is to focus on what can be controlled in this present moment. The athlete can resist, or flow; can stay angry, or find acceptance and a positive mind-set. Countless psychophysiological studies have been done to show the correlation between moods and physiological responses in the body. For example, Simpson et al. (2008) measured salivary cortisol levels with positive and negative mood states. The authors found increased levels of cortisol with negative mood states and decreased levels of cortisol with positive mood states. Entire academic departments, medical specialties, and publications are devoted to biological psychology. It is beyond the scope of this project to offer an extensive literature review on the findings in this area of inquiry. Suffice it to say that the link between psychology and biology, between the mental and the physical, between thoughts, emotions, and physiological processes, is undeniable. Stress releases cortisol, and cortisol breaks down muscle tissue and prolongs recovery. So staying positive and mentally focused on recovery will facilitate the return to activity.

In *Running Within,* Jerry Lynch and Warren Scott write, "The most prevalent response to running injury or illness is panic; the most essential ingredient for healing and recovery is hope" (p. 152). Lynch and Scott report on various national teams using visualization techniques to heal injuries more quickly than even doctors predicted. Athletes who visualize what is happening in their body have been reported to heal their injuries faster than those who did not practice visualization techniques. Visualization also helps athletes feel more in control of what is happening to them and less a victim of their circumstances. This feeling of control helps shift a negative mood into a positive one and thus sets the body on the trajectory of healing. Reducing stress in the body through a positive mood state enables the body to heal faster by increasing blood flow, decreasing heart rate and blood pressure, and limiting the release of catabolic hormones.

There is also much that can be done regarding nutrition to facilitate recovery, particularly in the realm of reducing inflammation. The connection between nutrition and healing is paramount and well documented.

Nutrition

It is vital to an athlete's success that the workouts and the recovery days are fueled both during injured periods and healthier times. Endurance athletes who are prone to exercise dependence, particularly for weight-loss reasons, may not fuel adequately if a workout is missed. It is perhaps logical or tempting to think that an off day or a missed workout day warrants restricting calories. And to a certain extent, this is not entirely false. It is, however, dangerous for an athlete to restrict so much that the ability to recover from the previous workout is compromised due to a fear of consuming calories without an accompanying workout. Even on an off day, a 120-pound athlete should be taking in close to 1,800 kcal, which is only 200 kcal less than the daily average recommendations. Restricting too much is dangerous and detrimental to subsequent performance.

This is not going to be a treatise on nutrition; there are many quality texts already in print that cover sport nutrition. However, I would be negligent to not at least mention nutrition in this work. The key contribution of my research is that the more athletes exercise to reach a certain body ideal, the higher their incidence for exercise dependence. Exercise is only one component of that equation, however. In striving to reach a particular body type, nutrition is another key component. Thus I offer some guidelines and recommendations for endurance athletes. As a certified sport nutritionist through the International Society of Sport Nutrition, I am able to speak with authority on the nutritional needs of athletes.

While I am not an advocate of counting calories, I approach this nutrition section in terms of calories to drive home the point that even on off days, athletes still need to eat. Knowledge of an athlete's weight is necessary to plan how many calories should be taken in. Starting with weight, calculate basal metabolic rate (BMR), or how many calories the body needs to stay alive. The Mifflin-St. Joer Equation is a highly reliable equation that takes into account weight, height, and age to calculate BMR. The only drawback to the Mifflin-St. Joer Equation is that it does not take into account body fat or lean muscle mass. This can lead to underestimating the needs of those with low body fat and overestimating the needs of those with higher body fat. However, the equation is a valuable tool to begin to understand the caloric needs of athletes.

To calculate BMR using the Mifflin-St. Jeor Equations:

Male: BMR = 10 x weight (kg) + 6.25 x height (cm) − 5 x age (yrs) +5

Female: BMR $= 10x$ weight (kg) $+ 6.25$ x height (cm) $- 5$ x age (yrs) - 161

With this information of BMR, factor in the calories burned through daily living, walking to work, school, etc. Here's how:

1. If suffering from an injury or taking some prolonged time off of exercise, multiply your BMR by 1.2. The resulting number will be an estimate of daily caloric intake.

2. If in an off season or exercising three days per week, multiply your BMR by 1.375. The resulting number will be an estimate of daily caloric intake, averaging out the three days of exercise per week over the course of seven days.

3. If training five days per week, multiply your BMR by 1.55.

4. If training six or seven days per week, multiply your BMR by 1.725.

5. If training six or seven days per week with double sessions, multiply BMR by 1.9.

The above estimates average weekly training volume, so missing one day of training does not necessitate deviating drastically from the above formulas. To avoid major shifts in energy consumption, it is best to average weekly calories burned instead of daily caloric expenditure. As one nutritionist informed me, "Nutrition is not accounting; the books don't close at the end of the night." And that is why it is a better idea to use the above equations based on weekly estimates than to adjust caloric consumption on a daily basis.

Many argue that "calories in equals calories out," and they are right, to a certain extent. What this concise axiom of nutrition means is that body mass changes as a direct result of the balance or imbalance of the equation "calories in $=$ calories out." If more calories are consumed (calories in) than burned (calories out), the result is weight gain. If more calories are burned (calories out) than consumed (calories in), this results in weight loss. So, a deviation from this equation, "calories in $=$ calories out," results in either an addition or depletion of body mass.

This is a simplified understanding of what is happening in the body. Remember, the books don't close at midnight. I advocate for calories in = calories out over the course of a weekly average, *not* a daily average. If a workout is missed, one may reason that there are no calories out, therefore there should be no calories in. That is a problematic and incorrect assumption. The athlete still needs calories to fuel basic life function. Just because one ran three hours yesterday and is not running today doesn't mean one shouldn't eat today. The body is still burning fuel to recover from the three-hour run completed yesterday and to repair the muscle breakdown from the previous day's effort. Very interesting research has been done with burn victims who are inactive and restricted to bed rest all day. Their caloric needs are as high, if not higher than, endurance athletes training one to three hours per day. Recovery and repair take energy, and that energy needs to come in the form of food. Thus, appropriate nutrition is necessary. I emphasize that severely restricting calories on an off day will sabotage the quality of a workout on subsequent days and compromise recovery between efforts. Instead, it is wiser to use weekly averages to calculate caloric needs instead of daily ones.

Nutrition is a key component of recovery, and fueling workouts is very important for athletes. Exercise addicts may hold faulty assumptions about caloric needs based on a missed workout, and this is a fallacy and only contributes to the incidence of underrecovery and overtraining.

Cross-training

There are a number of reasons why an athlete might miss a workout; whatever the cause, it's time to improvise. This is maybe hard to do when a rigid and methodical workout schedule is followed, but here is an opportunity to take a step back and reevaluate the big picture. One can still survive a day without a workout, and that doesn't mean that one is going to gain ten pounds and therefore shouldn't eat. I have already established that. What it does mean is that a more creative look at the surroundings is indicated, and one is challenged to figure out how else to stay active, even if it's not precisely what is prescribed on the schedule.

If the athlete is suffering from an injury and cannot train, perhaps he/she will try water running. I have many athletes train for marathons and triathlons with deep-water running. It is an excellent workout, trust me; one can feel sweat in the pool if working hard enough. Cycling, depending on the injury, can be another alternative. Hiking or walking with the kids or the dog is another opportunity to be outside, spend time with the family, and remain active, albeit at a lower intensity than accustomed to. Put the kids in the trailer behind the bike and take a spin around the neighborhood. Capitalize on the opportunity to meld time with family, get the dog some exercise, and move around. A missed workout can be a wonderful opportunity to multitask and share passion for activity and the outdoors with others who are not quite at your level. Go with it.

Another alternative is yoga. Yoga focuses on developing core strength, which is crucial for injury prevention. It also increases flexibility and helps to develop total body strength, eliminating any weak links in the kinesthetic chain which often lead to injury as well.

I find yoga to be the cheapest therapy on the market. While some therapists charge up to $150 for a fifty-minute session, I have never paid over $20 for an hour yoga class, and I have gotten a lot more out of my yoga. Yoga challenges us to sit inside ourselves, to be present with our thoughts and emotions, to connect the mind with the body through the breath. There is no better way to bring training and racing to the next level than to become more aware of your body. And there is no better way to heal old wounds, be they physical, emotional, or psychological, than to really be with them and not distract yourself from them, not to stuff them down with food or bury them with tasks and obligations. Really sitting with that stuff is the only way to heal it. Just like recognizing and acknowledging the five steps of the grieving process is the only way to move through to acceptance, the same holds true with old emotional, physical, and psychological baggage. And yoga really helps to make us sit with our "stuff" with the hopes of being able to move through it, to let it go, and to heal.

Mediation/Visualization

Yoga also teaches the techniques of meditation—the tools to sit and be mindful and be present. If one is unable to train, try to meditate. Healing the body from injury and addiction through mental practices has been studied for decades.. If one doesn't have ninety minutes for a run or ride, finding ten minutes to sit and meditate seem more doable. This will help bring the body into balance and alignment. The athlete won't get the cardiovascular benefits of increasing heart rate, won't get the physiological benefits of teaching the body to utilize fat more efficiently as a fuel source, and won't increase lactate threshold, but he/she will be able to reduce cortisol levels, decrease resting heart rate, increase healthy circulating blood and lymphatic fluid, and find peace and calm in the interrupted routine of missing a workout.

It is hard to "just sit," but I encourage a trial "run." What is most difficult for an athlete is often what is needed the most. Many athletes know very well how to add one more thing and push themselves beyond the limits; after all, that is what athletics is all about. Meditation can push athletes beyond personal limits as well in a very different way, in a way that regrounds and recenters the person. The benefits will prove invaluable in the next training session and the next race day performance. Not only will the body be more balanced and healthy, the athlete will also have practiced the mental clarity to focus and push through mental barriers, which often is the limiting factor in competition. It is not the physical barriers, but the mental ones that limit potential. There is no better illustration of this than the breaking of the four-minute mile.

It was thought that no human could run a mile faster than four minutes; after all, it had never been done before. On May 6, 1954, Roger Bannister broke the four-minute mile. Six weeks later on June 21, John Landy bettered Bannister's sub-four-minute time by over one second. By the end of 1956, a total of nine runners had broken through the four-minute barrier. Training innovations, while continually improving, do not account for the rapid succession of runners running faster than thought humanly possible. Instead, the mental barrier had been broken. Bannister proved that running a mile in under four minutes was possible. By eliminating disbelief, the possibility and potential for others to achieve this record became imaginable. Physically, these runners were perhaps always able to achieve the feat, but knowing that it was possible, they were able to eliminate thoughts that held them back and were able to push through and actualize their potential.

How many times does one think "this is hard" or "I want to walk" and then stop running or decrease the pace? While certainly there are physiological factors that affect training and racing, it is thinking about the effort that ultimately affects the performance. In fact, St. Clair Gibson, Lambert et. al (2001) argue convincingly that an athlete's fatigue level is centrally governed. Through self-talk, processed in the brain, an athlete perceives a workout or effort level as more or less fatiguing based on thoughts concerning the effort itself. It is not the accumulation of lactate and the mitochondrial density that determines levels of fatigue; it is an athlete's thoughts concerning a workout and the associated sensations of the workout that ultimately dictate levels of fatigue, according to research conducted by St. Clair Gibson, Lambert et al.

If the athlete gives up mentally, the race is over; mentally, if one commits to push through, then one can reach new levels in performance. I know athletes are mentally committed to training; my research highlights the fact that there is a distinct Ironman mentality. An athlete has the potential to use that mentality to focus on positive coping skills to make it through an off day. The athlete knows how to commit, so instead of committing to being angry, resentful, and pissed off, commit to focusing on all that can be done with the opportunity for a break—meditate, sit with the self, learn to breathe, and be comfortable in yourself. Practice visualization; watch race-day success, watch the self pushing through the next hard workout, and visualize the tissues healing from the injury. See the off day as an opportunity to practice what is hard—flexibility. Learn to shift the mentality from a negative frame of mind to a positive one; this will not only help one make it through the day, one will emerge a healthier, more balanced individual and become much more pleasant to be around.

<u>Tips for the topsy-turvy day off</u>

1. Stay positive—see this as an opportunity to focus the time and energy on something else in life.

2. Don't restrict calories—this will negatively effect subsequent workouts and impede recovery.

3. Cross-train—try aquajogging, skiing, cycling, walking, roller-blading, or yoga. Be active and share love of activity and the outdoors with those who are not at a peak level of fitness.

4. Make workouts a team sport—put kids in the Tag-A-Long and take them on a "tour de parks" bike ride, stopping at all of the parks in the neighborhood. Go for a hike with the baby in the backpack. Take the pooch to the park.

5. Be flexible—it's okay to miss a workout every once in a while; it doesn't mean the end of the world. Take a step back from the compulsion and see there is more to living than doing each and every workout. Increasing stress and anxiety about missing a workout only serves to increase cortisol levels, and increased cortisol levels negatively affect recovery. So stay positive and know that life happens; one cannot micromanage each and every aspect of daily existence to ensure that absolutely every workout gets accomplished. That's okay. Look at the big picture and breathe.

6. Meditate—sit with the self, feel one's breath, calm the cells, and augment recovery for subsequent workouts with this therapeutic practice.

7. Visualize—see the self recovering more rapidly from injury or illness. Visualize pushing through the next hard workout. Envision successful completion of the next race. Use the off day to train mental skills while physical skills get to rest. Research shows that neural pathways are sharpened as a result of visualization. So even if one can't get out there and "do it," one can "imagine it" and will be preparing better for when one can get out there to "do it."

Chapter 6: Bringing It All Together for Optimal Existence

All too often, exercise is celebrated as an admirable endeavor. However, it is perhaps the case that others should not actually laud one's addiction. We don't celebrate the tenacity of the drunk at the bar, or the commitment and dedication of the addicted gambler. Nor do we praise the success of an anorexic who weighs eighty pounds. These are unhealthy behaviors, and they are widely recognized as such. Exercise, while it certainly has the potential to be a very healthy outlet for stress, a wonderful way to enjoy the outdoors, and a method of maintaining a healthy weight and cardiovascular system, also has the potential to subsume an individual, to ruin marriages, and to compromise health, both physically and mentally, and it is not often enough recognized as such. The potential for taking a healthy activity too far is all too present for endurance athletes, and intervention is paramount to healing and restoring balance.

Onlookers may find the completion of an Ironman a lost endeavor, and "outsiders" may find an athlete's commitment to completing a 100-mile UltraMarathon impressive, but the story is perhaps more complicated than the simple accomplishments themselves. Loved ones and friends likely feel the effects of the addicted individual's tendencies to prioritize training over everything else. Spouses and children alike conceivably bear witness to the addict's behavior of training through injury, his/her inability to take a rest day, and or his/her moodiness and irritability if and when a workout session is missed.

The cycle continues until there is recognition, until there is intervention. As long as these accomplishments are celebrated uncritically, intervention will never happen. However, when athletes begin the conversation, admitting that a healthy activity can be taken too far, when the addiction is named, the healing process begins. Make no mistake, it is possible to run 100 miles and race Ironman races *without* being an exercise addict. The EDQ was sensitive enough to discern addicts from nonaddicts, even within an Ironman population. It is the attitude with which one approaches one's training that determines the level of addiction—*not* the participation in the activity itself.

Consuming alcohol does not make one an alcoholic, rather it is the quantity, frequency, and behaviors surrounding alcohol consumption that constitute the addictive behavior. The same is true with exercise. For too long now, exercise has not been viewed as a potentially addictive behavior; it has been exempt from the list of addictive substances. Exercise needs to be viewed just as any other addictive substance. The repercussions of exercise addiction are just as damaging as any other addiction. Those who suffer from exercise addiction impair their physical and mental health and their ability to effectively relate with others. They suffer from ruined relationships, debilitating overuse injuries, and anxiety and depression. While pursuing "health" perchance, they are embodying the antithesis. As coaches, as mental health practitioners, as loved ones, and as athletes, it is imperative for us to recognize these behavioral patterns and intervene.

How to Recognize an Addiction

What constitutes addiction?
- Is there an addiction to exercise because of a desire to race? No.
- Because one wants to better the previous performance? No.
- Is training an addiction because the invested time and energy to achieve one's potential on race day was the focus? Certainly not.

I do not profess to make the snap judgment that one is and one is not an addict. I hear the counterargument resonating in my ears that "it takes dedication and a singular focus to succeed." And while I agree with that, it takes a singular focus to work hard *and* to recover hard. Addicts don't recover; they can't take a day off, and thus impede their own ability to succeed. This work does not lambaste all highly competitive and highly achieving athletes to label them as addicts. Instead it brings awareness to some potentially problematic patterns of behavior, for age groupers and elites alike, behaviors that can become all consuming and spiral out of control, leading to mental and physical ailments as well as interpersonal impediments (read: divorce). It is not the caliber or success of the athlete that constitutes his/her level of addiction; it is the attitude with which he/she approaches training. How often does the athlete resent training and look forward to the taper week just to make the race history? The athlete starts to become antsy during taper week, thinking about not burning enough calories to justify eating the big meal, or three meals in one day. The athlete arrives at race day, somewhat anxious about performance, second guessing, and wondering what motivated registering for the race in the first place. But toeing the starting line often quells prerace anxieties, and one starts to get curious and excited to lay it out on the line to see how this newfound fitness, these weeks of training, will do come race time. It's like taking a new car for a spin—how is the body going to perform? The athlete is out there racing, having fun, sort of- admittedly an obtuse definition of "fun." It's fun to push beyond thinking of personal limitations and to know what is possible from deep down. At some point during the race, thoughts may sound like, "Why am I doing this? Why pay money to do this? Remember, never do this again." And yet, as one crosses that finish line and within moments, minutes, hours, days (not even days typically), one's thoughts change to: "Is going faster possible? When's the next one?" And the cycle starts again. The athlete may feel lost without a training plan, without a goal race to focus around. One craves the freedom at the end of a build to go out with buddies, to not think about the 5:30 a.m. alarm, and yet when the opportunity arises for some downtime, the addicted athlete doesn't know how to handle it. Does this sound familiar?

Let's break it down.

1) Are there increased levels of anxiety when there is no race on the calendar?

Training can serve as a very convenient coping strategy to mask underlying issues. Without a goal race on the calendar and a training plan to organize the day, addicts no longer have a mask to hide behind. Training is no longer a distraction, and instead whatever was motivating the addiction comes to the surface, and that can be very challenging.

What motivates one to organize the desk or the kitchen when something in life feels out of control? While one can't get a handle on the larger issue, one can control the contents of the desk and the Tupperware—and somehow, that helps in its own way. One doesn't have to be an obsessive-compulsive individual, but in that moment, cleaning and organizing serves as a distraction from the larger issue at hand, and it offers a sense of stability and control when one is otherwise feeling a bit ungrounded.

Training plans and goal races can serve the very same purpose. They can stand in as orderly events when everything else in life feels a little unwieldy. Executing a training plan is often easier than looking at deeper, more complicated problems at hand. Exercise, thus, can be used as a stand-in object, just as cleaning and organizing can—even for the nonobsessive-compulsive individual.

2) Are there depression symptoms that training covers up?

Exercise does release endorphins, which can increase mood levels. Thus exercise can be used as a behavioral mood enhancement or mood stabilizer in addition to, or in place of, pharmaceuticals. Exercise can also externalize some of the internal angst an individual might be feeling. Just as cutting makes physical and tangible the psychological and emotional turmoil an individual may feel, pushing oneself physically can serve to transfer internal pain to external discomfort. Running all-out mile repeats, pushing up steep climbs, and physically feeling the limitations of the body, the burn of the muscle, can take one out of one's head and place one firmly in the materiality of the body. Focusing on muscle pain and on the top of a steep climb, or the stopwatch, is often easier than wrestling with larger-than-life questions of happiness. Such physical challenges place one firmly in the present moment and become all consuming, leaving no space for deliberating on a tough issue at work or home. Physical pain or discomfort elicited through tough interval workouts or all-out racing can serve as a distraction from emotional pain, but it is just that—a distraction—and serves only to mask whatever lies under the surface.

3) Does the athlete engage in "secret" training or do more than the coach puts on the training plan?

If the athlete is unable to take a day off or goes against the coach's orders, this is a very clear sign of exercise addiction. A close look at one's relationship to exercise is strongly recommended, as it has likely shifted from healthy to unhealthy.

4) Does the athlete "up the ante" each time and try for longer and longer distances?

This is known as the tolerance effect, and it is easily identifiable in drug addicts and alcoholics. Where once four beers caused intoxication, now it takes twelve. Addicts who use drugs increase their dosage in the attempt to reach the same high. When exercise is the drug of choice, goal events seem to grow in length and proportion.

There is a statistical correlation between exercise addiction scores and one's own motivation for training, namely the desire to alter one's body into a leaner version of oneself—and not for the purpose of racing faster, but instead for aesthetic purposes. Specifically, the more an athlete is influenced by social attitudes towards appearances, the more likely they are to be exercise dependent. This leads to the fifth and final tough question for identifying addictive tendencies.

5) Is the athlete controlled by the calories in/calories out continuum?

Does one restrict calories on off days? Count calories and abstain from eating when caloric expenditure does not warrant intake? Keep in mind, an anorexic is not healed when he/she begins eating only to engaging in hours of activity at the gym. Sure, he/she manipulates one side of the equation, "energy in" (by eating more), but the "calories out" portion of the equation increases as well; this is not healing, this is bait and switch. The equation is still winning, is still in control.

The athlete can recognize anorexia and bulimia as a problematic pattern of behavior, and yet when the very same pattern of behavior is executed through exercise, it is too often celebrated as an impressive endeavor. Exercise bulimia is recognized in mental health circles, but it is not often recognized in athletic populations.

6) Take the Exercise Dependence Questionnaire in Appendix A to measure personal levels of exercise dependence.

The EDQ is sensitive enough to isolate dependence patterns even among endurance athletes, since not all Ironman athletes score in the pathological range on the EDQ, and yet some did. Thus this testing tool seems appropriate for endurance athletes who train one to twenty hours per week and follow a training plan.

This work is a resource for mental health practitioners, for coaches, and, most importantly, for athletes themselves. It is time to take a close look at the growing popularity of marathons and triathlons and unpack what is going on behind the scenes. Twelve million athletes participated in triathlons in 2009. This is an 11% increase in participation in one year. The Sporting Goods Manufacturers Association is reporting a 51.4% increase in participation in triathlons since 2007. While this is a celebrated fact for the sport of triathlon and the manufacturers of sporting goods, I read this statistic with trepidation. Are endurance athletes rapidly at a tipping point—a la Gladwell—for something simmering under the surface? Until athletes, coaches, and mental health practitioners probe deeper in the motivations of endurance athletes, the answer will never be known.

Healing addictions, living a balanced life

Maybe exercise began as a benign and healthy outlet, and now it rules—the dog is no longer wagging the tail, the tail is wagging the dog. Perhaps the feeling of *having* to train or not feel okay, feeling one's mood is off, being unpleasant to be around, mean the athlete is controlled by the addiction, rather than controlling it. Evaluate that.

What is the goal? What is the motivation? Why train? If the answers look a certain way, proceed cautiously, and know there are tendencies that indicate addiction.

Keep in mind that identifying an issue is the first step to recovery—that is what this book hopes to accomplish. For many athletes, the words of the triathletes I interviewed will resonate. If that is the case, I do hope there is a recognition that what your friends see as a laudable endeavor may actually be much more complex than that. The great news is: change is possible. The athlete can sit with whatever exercise is covering up—is masking—and he/she can work on that piece from the inside out.

Change is not about buying a book and "fixing" the problem from the outside. It is instead about taking a close look at the motivations behind the training. Consider the difficult questions that training obscures. Seeking answers as to why exercise is a means for distraction and deciding what the athlete is distancing himself/herself from are additional questions. It is not sufficient to substitute one addiction for another—albeit, admittedly, there are seemingly more "functional" and less "functional" addictions—running versus methamphetamines, for example. But as this work has shown, addiction is addiction—and there are alternatives to opt out of the addictive pattern, to heal what simmers below the surface fueling the addiction in the first place. Exercise, as the substance of addiction, is more socially accepted than drugs or alcohol, and it is a clever and covert way of hiding addiction—as it can be couched in "training" for longer and longer endurance events. Exercise addiction, however, is still problematic for the mental, physical, and emotional health of the individual who suffers from the addiction.

It is from an inquiry into my own behaviors that this research emerged. I know signs of exercise addiction, because I am an exercise addict. My subjectivity enables me to ask the hard questions, to use my own lived experience as a launching point from which to investigate further into the burgeoning field of exercise addiction. As an endurance athlete, I wanted to dig further.

Personally, I know the tactics that addicts use to substantiate their unhealthy behavior. I come to this work from a place of self-inquiry. I can answer affirmatively to each and every one of the six questions above. I'm training six hours today to get ready for an upcoming race—and there's always an upcoming race. Athletes use the races to justify the addiction, to mask the problem. The athlete addict ups the ante, the races get longer and longer. What began as a journey into "I wonder if I can run a marathon" quickly turned into "I bet I could run 100 miles." I began with a marathon, then two, then an Ironman, then two—and it wasn't long until I was running 100-mile races. One day my mother remarked, "I never thought I would say this, but I wish you would 'just' run a marathon!"

I found marathon running through an unhealthy relationship with the "calories in, calories out" continuum. If I were expending more calories out, then I would lose weight faster. And thus began my downward spiral into exercise addiction. It was a clever way to mask an eating disorder, but I only ended up fooling myself. It has cost me relationships, it has caused me health issues, and it has certainly affected my mental health and happiness.

I sought healing through academic inquiry, and I continue to navigate my own way through this tricky addiction as an endurance athlete and as a coach. I am cognizant of my behavioral patterns, of my bouts with recovery and relapse. And, luckily, I have a wonderful support system whose members do not endorse my addictive habits. They endorse me, they love me, but they are the first ones to say "good for you" when I drop down from a 50-miler to a 25-miler in the middle of a race. They encourage me to listen to my body when it is sending me signals loud and clear. They advise me to sit with my stuff when I tell them it's easier to train for a 100-mile race than to *not* train for a 100-mile race. They make me look in the mirror and see what I have done to myself in the vain attempt to look like the supermodels I will never be—I am five-foot-two, after all—and, as one coach commented, "built like a shot-putter."

That's me, highest bench press and slowest mile time on my Division I lacrosse team. And yet I took this stocky build and ran with it. Literally, ran 100 miles in Leadville, ran a marathon at the end of a 112-mile bike ride in Kona, ran through the streets of Boston year after year. And

I continue to run, to run away, and to run towards something other than what is, right now. And yet sitting with what is, right now, is the solution, is the healing process. That is why yoga and meditation are so fundamental to countering the addiction. Addictions serve as tools to resist the present moment for what it is. They serve to distract one from the task at hand. What if the addicted athlete embraces what is right now? What would happen then? That person would perhaps loosen his/her grasp on the addiction. He/she would begin to get in touch with the inner self, the true self behind the one that simply executes the training plan, the authentic self behind the mask of training and racing.

For too long I have hid behind the races, the training plans, and the next event and longer event. I didn't know who the self was without the events, and I am still struggling to find that person. As it happens, the universe presents us with lessons just in the moment we need to learn them. As I finish up this book, I do so with my arm in a sling, two broken bones in my shoulder, and three staples in my head. I suffered a bike accident and now am forced to follow my own advice. I have had to pull out of two races and one yoga clinic. I have never taken more than two days off of running, and I rarely take one full day of inactivity; yoga is how I fill my recovery days. And yet, now I have no choice. I cannot run, I cannot ride, I cannot do yoga. I can sit with my injury and try to stay positive, try to learn the lessons that are meant to be learned (watch out for potholes and gravel when descending on a twisty mountain pass—that's only one of them).

Other lessons include getting in touch with who I am when I am not training—for training has been so central to my identity for so long. In fact, the only plans I had for the holiday weekend over which I was injured included riding, running, and yoga. Without those activities, my weekend was suddenly devoid of plans. I had to fill it with movies and spending time with friends. This is new for me, and yet so enlightening— I am a person even if I don't run for four hours. I am still a human not atop my bike or on my yoga mat. I haven't disintegrated yet, and while it's been challenging to reframe and refocus how I spend my time, it is enlightening to see that there are alternatives to enjoying the day that don't involve extensive activity. Now that may sound comical to the sedentary population, but as I left the hospital on the Friday of a holiday weekend, I was seriously wondering how people spent their time if they weren't running or riding all day—as that was how I had envisioned the weekend playing out.

It is infinitely easier to write about these issues than to embody and enact the solutions, I know. And yet that is precisely what I am challenged to do right. If I can do it, so can any addicted athlete—at least I can promise to try. Healing both physically and emotionally requires accepting the present moment as it is. I have written these words in the past, and now it is incumbent upon me to stand behind them—staples and all. The broken bones will heal, the staples will come out, and then who will I be? I have the option of dropping right back into my addictive patterns, *and* I have the opportunity to make a change, to find more balance, more space, and more health in the endeavors I pursue, be they 100-mile races or acts of daily living. Healing will happen. The physical healing is the easy part; it's the emotional healing that takes more attention and effort. I will heal and I will find balance, because I am committed to it.

I offer this work for every other endurance athlete who seeks healing and balance in his/her life; who has toed the line of addiction and rationalized his/her way to the other side. This book can be a life raft back to civilization, to a world apart from constant calorie counting and continual movement, back to a world of balance and belonging.

Appendix A

Exercise Dependence Questionnaire (EDQ)
Ogden, Veale, and Summers (1997)
Age_____ Sex_____

I exercise _____/week (this included yoga, Pilates, lifting, stretching, as well as biking, running, and swimming workouts).

Below are a series of statements that people have used to describe their attitudes to exercise. Please rate each of the statements by circling the appropriate number for how much it describes your attitude to your own exercise over the past month (in season/out of season). Please use the following scale.

Strongly Disagree Strongly Agree
1	2	3	4	5	6	7

1. My level of exercising makes me tired at work. _____
2. After an exercise session I feel happier about life. _____
3. If I cannot exercise I feel irritable. _____
4. The rest of my life has to fit in around my exercise. _____
5. After an exercise session I feel less anxious. _____
6. I exercise to look attractive. _____
7. I sometimes miss time at work to exercise. _____
8. After an exercise session I feel that I am a better person. _____
9. If I cannot exercise I feel agitated. _____
10. I exercise to meet other people. _____
11. I hate not being able to exercise. _____
12. I exercise to keep me occupied. _____
13. If I cannot exercise, I feel I cannot cope with life. _____
14. I exercise to control my weight (I exercise to eat what I want).
_____

Strongly Disagree Strongly Agree

| 1 | 2 | 3 | 4 | 5 | 6 | 7 |

15. I have little energy for my partner, family, and friends._____

16. Being thin (lean) is the most important thing in my life. _____

17. I feel guilty about the amount I exercise. _____

18. I exercise to be healthy. _____

19. After an exercise session I feel thinner. _____

20. My level of exercise has become a problem. _____

21. I make a decision to exercise (race) less, but I cannot stick to it. _____

22.) I exercise for the same amount of time each week (in and out of season). _____

23. After an exercise session I feel more positive about myself. _____

24. My weekly pattern of exercise is repetitive. _____

25. My pattern of exercise interferes with my social life. _____

26. I exercise to feel fit. _____

27. My exercising is running my life. _____

28. I exercise to prevent heart disease and other illnesses._____

29. If I cannot exercise I miss the social life. _____

Scoring: Add up the total of your score, if your sum total is over 116, you are above the cutoff score for healthy exercise.

Appendix B: Sociocultural Attitudes Towards Appearance Scale (SATAQ-3R)

The thirty-eight-item Sociocultural Attitudes Towards Appearance Questionnaire 3 Revised edition (SATAQ-3R) subscales include pressures, importance, social comparison, and internalization (TV/magazine, comparison, and athletics).

This scale is scored from 1 to 5: definitely disagree, somewhat disagree, neither disagree nor agree, somewhat agree, and definitely agree.

Importance

1. TV programs are an important source of information about fashion and "being attractive."
2. TV commercials are an important source of information about fashion and "being attractive."
3. Music videos on TV are an important source of information about fashion and "being attractive."
4. Magazine articles are an important source of information about fashion and "being attractive."
5. Magazine advertisements are an important source of information about fashion and "being attractive."
6. Pictures in magazines are an important source of information about fashion and "being attractive."
7. Movies are an important source of information about fashion and "being attractive."
8. Movie stars are an important source of information about fashion and "being attractive."

9. Famous people are an important source of information about fashion and "being attractive."

Pressures

1. I've felt pressure from TV or magazines to lose weight.

2. I've felt pressure from TV or magazines to look pretty.

3. I've felt pressure from TV or magazines to be thin.

4. I've felt pressure from TV or magazines to have a perfect body.

5. I've felt pressure from TV or magazines to diet.

6. I've felt pressure from TV or magazines to exercise.

7. I've felt pressure from TV or magazines to change my appearance.

Internalization—TV/Magazine

1. I would like my body to look like the people who are on TV.

2. I would like my body to look like the models who appear in magazines.

3. I would like my body to look like the people who are in movies.

4. I wish I looked like the models in music videos.

5. I try to look like the people on TV.

6. I try to look like the people in music videos.

Internalization—Athlete

1. I wish I looked as athletic as the people in magazines.

2. I wish I looked as athletic as sports stars.

3. I try to look like sports athletes.

Internalization—Comparison

1. I compare my body to the bodies of TV and movie stars.

2. I compare my appearance to the appearance of TV and movie stars.

3. I compare my body to the bodies of people who appear in magazines.

4. I compare my appearance to the appearance of people in magazines.

Awareness

1. Clothes look better on people who are attractive.

2. Clothes look better on people who are thin.

3. Clothes look better on people who have an athletic body.

4. Attractive people are better liked than unattractive people.

5. People who are thin are better looking than people who are overweight.

6. People who have an athletic body are better looking.

7. Physically fit people are more attractive.

8. Good-looking people are more successful.

9. Attractive people are happier.

Scoring: Add up scores in each subsection to identify categorically what influences you the most.

Works Cited

Adams, J., and R. Kirby. 1998. Exercise dependence: A review of its manifestation, theory, and measurement. *Sports Medicine Training and Rehabilitation, 8*, 265–276.

Adams, J., T. Miller, and R. Kraus. 2003. Exercise dependence: Diagnostic and therapeutic issues for patients in psychotherapy. *Journal of Contemporary Psychotherapy, 33*(2), 93–107.

Adkins, E., and P. Keel. 2005. Does "excessive" or "compulsive" best describe exercise as a symptom of bulimia nervosa? *International Journal of Eating Disorders, 38*, 24–29.

Agliata, D., and S. Tantleff-Dunn. 2004. The impact of media exposure on male's body image. *Journal of Social and Clinical Psychology, 23*(1), 7–22.

American Psychiatric Association. 1994. *Diagnostic and statistical manual of mental disorders* (fourth edition). Washington, DC.

Anshel, M. H. 1991. A psychobehavioral analysis of addicted versus non-addicted male and female exercisers. *Journal of Sport Behavior, 14*, 145–154.

Aravich, P. F. 1996. Adverse effects of exercise stress and restricted feeding in the rat: Theoretical and neurobiological considerations. In *Activity anorexia theory, research, and treatment*, ed. W. F. Epling and W. D. Pierce, 81–97. Hillsdale, NJ: Erlbaum.

Babbitt, B. 2003. *25 years of the Ironman Triathlon world championship*. Adelaide, Australia: Meyer and Meyer Sport.

Bacon, J. G., K. E. Scheltema, and B. E. Robinson. 2001. Fat phobia scale revisited: The short form. *International Journal of Obesity, 25*, 252–257.

Bamber, D., I. Cockerill, and D. Carroll. 2000. The pathological status of exercise dependence. *British Journal of Sports Medicine, 34*, 125–132.

------. 2002. Diagnostic criteria for exercise dependence in women. *British Journal of Sports Medicine, 37*, 393–400.

Bamber, D., I. Cockerill, S. Rodgers, and D. Carroll. 2003. Proposed diagnostic criteria for primary and secondary exercise dependence. *British Journal of Sports Medicine, 37,* 393–400.

Bamberger, M., ed. 2000. *Integrating quantitative and qualitative research in development projects.* Washington, DC: World Bank.

Beck, A. T., C. H. Ward, M. Mendelsohn, and J. Erbaugh. 1961. An inventory for measuring depression. *Archives of General Psychiatry, 4,* 561–571.

Bell, G., and B. Howe. 1988. Mood state profiles and motivations of triathletes. *Journal of Sport Behavior, 11*(20), 66–77.

Birke. L., and G. Vines. 1987. A sporting chance: The anatomy of destiny. *Women's Studies International Forum, 10*(4), 337–347.

Birrell, S., and N. Theberge. 1994. Feminist resistance and transformation in sport. In *Women and sport: Interdisciplinary perspectives*, ed. D. M. Costa and S. Guthrie, 361–376. Champaign, IL: Human Kinetics.

Black, R. 1991. Eating disorders among athletes: Current perspective. In *Eating disorders among athletes*, ed. D. R. Black, 1–10. Reston, VA: American Alliance for Health, Recreation, and Dance.

Blaydon, M., and K. Lindner. 2002. Eating disorders and exercise dependence in triathletes. *Eating Disorders, 10,* 49–60.

Blumenthal, J., L. O'Toole, and J. Chang. 1984. Is running an analogue of anorexia nervosa? An empirical study of obligatory running and anorexia nervosa. *Journal of the American Medical Association, 252*(4), 520–523.

Bordo, S. 1989. The body and the reproduction of femininity: A feminist appropriation of Foucault. In *Gender / body / knowledge: Feminist reconstructions of being and knowing*, ed. A. Jagger and S. Bordo, 13–33. New Brunswick, NJ: Rutgers University Press.

------. 1993. *Unbearable weight: Feminism, western culture, and the body*. Berkeley, CA: University of California Press.

------. 1997. Reading the male body. In *Building bodies*, ed. P. Moore, 31–74. New Brunswick, NJ: Rutgers University Press.

Broocks, A., U. Schweiger, and K. M. Pirke. 1991. The influence of semi-starvation-induced hyperactivity on hypothalamic serotonin metabolism. *Psychology and Behavior. 50,* 385–388.

Bryman, A. 1988. *Quantity and quality in social research*. London: Routledge.

Buccinio, L. A. 1992. The construction and validation of the Running Dependence Inventory: Measurement of a heretofore elusive construct. *Dissertation Abstracts International, 53* (3-B), 1645.

Butler, J.(1990. *Gender trouble: Feminism and the subversion of identity*. New York: Routledge.

------. 1993. *Bodies that matter: On the discursive limits of "sex."* New York: Routledge.

------. 1997. *Excitable speech: A politics of the performative*. New York: Routledge.

Cahn, S. K. 1994. *Coming on strong: Gender and sexuality in twentieth-century women's sport*. Cambridge, MA: Harvard University Press.

Calogero, R., W. Davis, and J. Thomspon. 2004. The Sociocultural Attitudes Towards Appearance Questionnaire (SATAQ-3): Reliability and normative comparisons of eating disorder patients. *Body Image*, 1, 193-198.

Carmack, M., and R. Martens. 1979. Measuring commitment to running, a survey of runners' attitudes and mental states. *Journal of Sports Psychology, 1,* 25–42.

Chaouloff, F. 1989. Physical exercise and brain monoamines: A review. *Acta Physiologica Scandinavica, 137*, 1–13.

Chapman, C. L., and J. M. DeCastro. 1990. Running addiction: Measurements and associated psychological characteristics. *Journal of Sports Medicine and Physical Fitness, 30*, 283–290.

Cixous, H. 1976. The laugh of the medusa. *Signs, 1*(4), 875–893.

Clough, P., J. Shepherd, and R. Maughan. 1990. Motives for participation in recreational running. *Journal of Leisure Research, 21*, 297–309.

Cole, C. 1993. Resisting the cannon: Feminist cultural studies, sport, and technologies of the body. *Journal of Sport and Social Issues. 12,* 77–97.

Cook, J. 1992. *The triathletes: A season in the lives of four women in the toughest sport of all*. New York: St. Martin's Press.

Creswell, J. W. 2003. *Research design: Qualitative, quantitative, and mixed methods approaches* (second edition). Thousand Oaks, CA: Sage.

Creswell, J. W., and V. Plano Clark. 2007. *Designing and conducting mixed methods research.* Thousand Oaks, CA: Sage.

Crossman, J. 1987. Responses of competitive athletes to lay-off in training: Exercise addiction or psychological relief? *Journal of Sport Behavior, 10*(1), 28–38.

Davis, C., H. Brewer, and G. Ratusny. 1993. Behavioral frequency and psychological commitment: necessary concepts in the study of excessive exercising. *Journal of Behavioral Medicine, 16,* 611–628.

Davis, C., and J. Fox. 1993. Excessive exercise and weight preoccupation in women. *Addictive Behavior, 18,* 201–211.

Davis, C., S. Kennedy, E. Ralevski, M. Dionne, H. Brewer, C. Neitzert, and D. Ratusny. 1995. Obsessive compulsiveness and physical activity in anorexia nervosa and high-level exercising. *Journal of Psychosomatic Research, 39*(8), 967–976.

de Beauvoir, S. 1989. *The second sex.* New York: Vintage. (Original work published 1949.)

Derogatis, L. 1976. The SCL-90-R. Baltimore, MD: Clinical Psychometric Research.

DiGioacchino DeBate, R., H. Wethington, and R. Sargent. 2002a. Body size dissatisfaction among male and female triathletes. *Eating and Weight Disorders, 7*(4), 316–323.

------. 2002b. Subclinical eating disorder characteristics among male and female triathletes. *Eating and Weight Disorders, 7*(3), 210–220.

Duncan, M. C. 1994. The politics of women's body images and practices: Foucault, the panopticon, and *Shape* magazine. *Journal of Sport and Social Issues. 14*(1), 48–65.

Dworkin, S. L., and M. Messner. 1999. Just do … what? In *Revisioning gender*, ed. M. M. Ferree, J. Lorber, and B. Hess, 341–361. Thousand Oaks, CA: Sage.

Edwards, G., M. M. Gross, M. Keller, J. Moser, and R. Room. 1977. *Alcohol related disabilities.* Geneva, Switzerland: World Health Organization.

Fairburn, C. G., and S. J. Beglin. 1994. Assessment of eating disorders: Interview or self-report questionnaire? *International Journal of Eating Disorders, 16,* 363.

Fincher, R., and J. M. Jacobs. 1998. *Cities of difference.* New York: Guilford.

Firestone, S. 1970. *The dialectic of sex: The case for feminist revolution.* New York: Farrar, Straus, and Giroux.

Flax, J. 1990. *Thinking fragments: Psychoanalysis, feminism, and postmodernism in the contemporary west.* Berkeley, CA: University of California Press.

Foucault, M. 1980. *The history of sexuality: Volume I: An introduction.* Trans. R. Hurley. New York: Vintage Books, Random House.

Freud, S. 1930. *Civilization and its discontents.* New York: W. W. Norton.

Friedan, B. 1964. *The feminine mystique.* New York: Dell.

Garman, J. F., D. M. Hayduk, D. A. Crider, and M. M. Hodel. 2004. Occurrence of exercise dependence in a college-aged population. *Journal of American College Health*, 52(5), 221–228.

Garner, D. M., and P. E. Garfinkel. 1979. The Eating Attitudes Test: An index of symptoms of anorexia nervosa. *Psychological Bulletin*, 9, 273–279.

Garner, D. M., M. P. Olmsted, Y. Bohr, and P. E. Garfinkel. 1982. The Eating Attitudes Test: Psychometric features and clinical correlates. *Psychological Medicine, 12,* 871–878.

Garner, D., M. Olmsted, and J. Polivy. 1983. Development and validation of a multidimensional eating disorder inventory for anorexia nervosa and bulimia. *International Journal of Eating Disorders, 2*(2), 15–34.

Gilligan, C. 1993. *In a difference voice: Psychological theory and women's development.* Cambridge, MA: Harvard University Press.

Granskog, J. 1992. Tri-ing together: An exploratory analysis of the social networks of female and male triathletes. *Play and Culture,* 5(1), 76–91.

Griffiths, M. 1997. Exercise addiction: A case study. *Addiction Research,* 5(2), 161–168.

Grossman, A, 1985. Endorphins: "Opiates for the masses." *Medicine, Science, Sports, and Exercise, 17,* 101–105.

Grosz, E. 1994. *Volatile bodies: Toward a corporeal feminism*. Bloomington, IN: Indiana University Press.

Guttmann, A. 1991. *Women's sports: A history*. New York: Columbia University Press.

Halson, S., and A. Jeukendrup. 2004. Does overtraining exist? An analysis of overreaching and overtraining research. *Sports Medicine, 34*(14), 967–981.

Haraway, D. 1991. *Simians, cyborgs, and women: The reinvention of nature*. New York: Routledge.

Hargreaves, J. A. 1994. *Sporting females: Critical issues in the history and sociology of women's sport*. New York: Routledge.

Hathaway, S. R., and J. C. McKinley. 1948. *Minnesota Multiphasic Personality Inventory*. New York: Psychological.

Hauck, E., and J. Blumenthal. 1992. Obsessive and compulsive traits in athletes. *Sports Medicine, 14*, 215–227.

Hausenblas, H., and D. Symons Downs. 2002a. Exercise dependence: A systematic review. *Psychology of Sport and Exercise, 3*, 89–123.

------. 2002b..How much is too much? The development and validation of the Exercise Dependence Scale. *Psychology and Health. 17*(4), 387–404.

Heywood, L., and S. Dworkin. 2003 *Built to win: The female athlete as cultural icon*. Minneapolis, MN: University of Minnesota Press.

Hilliard, D. 1988. Finishers, competitors, and pros: A description and speculative interpretation of the triathlon scene. *Play and Culture, 1*, 300–313.

Huebner, H. F. 1993. *Endorphins, eating disorders, and other addictive behaviors*. New York: W. W. Norton.

Irigaray, L. 1985. *Speculum of the other woman*. Trans. G. C. Gill. New York: Cornell University Press.

Johnson, R. B., and A. J. Onweugbuzie. 2004. Mixed methods research: A research paradigm whose time has come. *Educational Researcher, 33*(7), 14–26.

Kessler, S., and W. McKenna. 1985. *Gender: An ethnomethodological approach*. Chicago: University of Chicago Press. (Original work published 1978.)

Kirby, K. 1996. Remapping subjectivity: Cartographic vision and the limits of politics. In *BodySpace: Destabilizing geographies of gender and sexuality*, ed. N. Duncan. New York: Routledge.

Knapp, C. 2003. *Appetites:Why women want*. New York: Counterpoint.

Kuscsik, N. 1977. The history of women's participation in the marathon. *Annals of the New York Academy of Sciences, 301,* 862–876.

Lal, J. 1996. Situating locations: The politics of self, identity, and "other" in living and writing the text. In *Dilemmas in feminist fieldwork*, ed. D. Wolf, 185–214. Boulder, CO: Westview.

Lawson, J. S., W. L. Marshall, and P. McGrath. 1979. The social self-esteem inventory. *Educational and Psychological Measurement, 39,* 803–811.

Lehmann, M. J., W. Lormes, A. Opitz-Gress, J. M. Steinacker, N. Netzer, C. Foster, and U. Gastmann. 1997. Training and overtraining: An overview and experimental results in endurance sports. *Journal of Sports Medicine and Physical Fitness. 37*(1), 7–17.

Lenskyj, H. 1990. Common sense and physiology: North American medical views on women and sport, 1890–1930. *Canadian Journal of History of Sport, 21*(1), 49–64.

Levenson, H. 1973. Multidimensional locus of control in psychiatric patients. *Journal of Consulting and Clinical Psychiatry, 41,* 397–404.

Lynch, J., and W. Scott. 1999. *Running within: A guide to mastering the body-mind-spirit connection of ultimate training and racing.* Champaign, IL: Human Kinetics.

Marchant, D., and A. Levy. 2005. Exercise dependence and fat phobia: Pilot data. *Journal of Sports Science, 23,* 1259–1262.

Marrazzi, M. A., and E. D. Luby. 1986. An auto-addiction opioid model of chronic anorexia nervosa. *International Journal of Eating Disorders, 5,* 191–208.

Masters, K. S., and M. J. Lambert. 1989. On gender comparison and construct validity: An examination of the commitment to running scale in a sample of marathon runners. *Journal of Sport Behavior, 12,* 196–202.

McDermott, B. 1979. Ironman. *Sports Illustrated.* May. 88-92.

Messner, M. A., and D. Sabo. 1990. *Sport, men and the gender order: Critical feminist perspectives*. Champaign, IL: Human Kinetics.

Mond, J., P. Hay, B. Rodgers, and C. Owen. 2006. An update on the definition of excessive exercise in eating disorder research. *International Journal of Eating Disorders*, *39*(2), 147–153.

Moore, P. L. 1997. Knowing bodies. In *Building bodies*, ed. P. Moore, 1–9. New Brunswick, NJ: Rutgers University Press.

Morgan, D. L. 1998. Practical strategies for combining qualitative and quantitative methods: Application to health research. *Qualitative Health Research, 8*(3), 362–376.

Morgan, W. P. 1979. Negative addiction in runners. *Physician and Sportsmedicine 7*(2), 57–70.

Morris, M., H. Steinberg, E. Sykes, and P. Salmon. 1990. Effects of temporary withdrawal from regular running. *Journal of Psychosomatic Research. 34*(5), 493–500.

Morse, J. M. 1991. Approaches to qualitative–quantitative methodological triangulation. *Nursing Research, 40,* 120–123.

Mrozek, D. 1987. The "Amazon" and the American "lady": Sexual fears of women as athletes. In *From "fair sex" to feminism: Sports and the socialization of women in the industrial and post-industrial eras*, ed. J. A. Mangan and R. J. Park, 282–298. Totowa, NJ: Frank Cass.

Murphy, R. 1990. *The body silent*. New York: W. W. Norton.

Nudelman, S., J. Rosen, and H. Leitenberg. 1988. Dissimilarities in eating attitudes, body image distortion, depression, and self-esteem between high-intensity male runners and women with bulimia nervosa. *International Journal of Eating Disorders, 7*(5), 625–634.

Ogden, J., D. Veale, and Z. Summers. 1997. The development and validation of the Exercise Dependence Questionnaire. *Addiction Research, 5*, 343–356.

Pasman, L., and J. Thompson. 1988. Body image and eating disturbance in obligatory runners, obligatory weight lifters and sedentary individuals. *International Journal of Eating Disorders. 7,* 759–769.

Pope, H. G., Jr., K. A. Phillips, and R. Olivardia. 2000. *The Adonis complex: The secret crisis of male body obsession*. New York: Free Press.

Reichardt, C. S., and S. F. Rallis, ed. 1994. *The qualitative–quantitative debate: New Perspectives.* San Francisco: Jossey-Bass.

Riley, D. 1988. *"Am I that name?" Feminism and the category of "women" in history.* Minneapolis: University of Minnesota Press.

Robinson, B. E., J. G. Bacon, and J. O'Reilly. 1993 Fat phobia: Measuring, understanding, and changing anti-fat attitudes. *International Journal of Eating Disorders, 14*(4), 467–480.

Rosenberg, M. 1979. *Conceiving the self.* New York: Basic Books.

Rossman, G. B., and B. L. Wilson. 1985. Numbers and words: Combining quantitative and qualitative methods in a single large-scale evaluation study. *Evaluation Review, 9*(5), 627–643.

Sachs, M. L., and D. Pargman. 1979. Running addiction: An in-depth interview examination. *Journal of Sport Behavior, 2*, 143–155.

------. 1984. *Running as therapy: An integrated approach.* Lincoln: University of Nebraska Press.

Samuels, E. 2002. Critical divides: Judith Butler's body theory and the question of disability. *National Women's Studies Association Journal, 14*(3), 58–76.

Scheper-Hughes, N., and M. Lock. 1987. The mindful body: A prolegomenon to future work in medical anthropology. *Medical Anthropology Quarterly, 1*, 6–41.

Shaulis, D. 1996. Women of endurance: Pedestriennes, marathoners, ultramarathoners, and others: Two hundred years of women and endurance. *Women in Sport and Physical Activity Journal, 5*(2), 1–27.

Simpson E. E. A., C. McConville, G. Rae, J. M. O'Connor, B. J. Stewart-Knox, C. Coudray, and J. J. Strain. 2008. Salivary cortisol, stress, and mood in healthy older adults: The Zenith study. *Biological Psychology*, 78 (1), pp. 1-9.

Slay, H., J. Hayaki, M. Napolitano, and K. Brownell. 1998. Motivations for running and eating attitudes in obligatory versus nonobligatory runners. *International Journal of Eating Disorders, 23*, 267–275.

Smolak, L., M. Levine, and K. Thompson. 2001. The use of Social Cultural Attitudes Towards Appearance Questionnaire with middle school boys and girls. *International Journal of Eating Disorders, 29*, 216–223.

140

Spelman, E. 1988. *Inessential woman: Problems of exclusion in feminist thought*. Boston: Beacon Press.

Spielberger, C. D., R. R. Gorsuch, and R. Lushene. 1970. *The State-Trait Anxiety Inventory (STAI) test manual*. Palo Alto, CA: Consulting Psychologists Press.

Sundgot-Borgen, J. 1993. Prevalence of eating disorders in elite female athletes. *International Journal of Sport Nutrition, 3*, 29–40.

------. 1999. Eating disorders among male and female elite athletes. *British Journal of Sports Medicine, 33,* 434.

Szabo, A., R. Frenkl, and A. Caputo. 1997. Relationships between addiction to running, commitment to running, and deprivation from running: A study on the Internet. *European Yearbook of Sport Psychology, 1*, 130–147.

Terry, A., A. Szabo, and M. Griffiths. 2004. The Exercise Addiction Inventory: A new brief screening tool. *Addiction Research and Theory, 12*(5), 489–499.

Thompson, J. K., and P. Blanton. 1987. Energy conservation and exercise dependence: A systematic arousal hypothesis. *Medicine and Science in Sports and Exercise, 19*, 91–99.

Thompson, J. K., P. van den Berg, M. Roehrig, A. Guarda, and L. J. Heinberg. 2004. The Sociocultural Attitudes Towards Appearance Scale-3. *International Journal of Eating Disorders, 35*, 293–304.

Thompson, R. A., and R. T. Sherman. 1993. *Helping athletes with eating disorders*. Champaign, IL: Human Kinetics.

Thoren, P., J. Floras, P. Hoffman, and D. Seals. 1990. Endorphins and exercise: Physiological mechanisms and clinical implications. *Medicine and Science in Sports and Exercise 22*(4), 417–428.

Urhausen, A., and W. Kindermann. 2002. Diagnosis of overtraining: What tools do we have? *Sports Medicine, 32*(2), 95–102.

Veale, C. 1987. Exercise dependence. *British Journal of Addiction, 82*, 735–740.

Vertinsky, P. 1994a. *The eternally wounded woman: Women, doctors, and exercise in the late nineteenth century*. Champaign: University of Illinois Press.

------. 1994b. Gender relations, women's history and sport history: A decade of changing enquiry, 1983–1993. *Journal of Sport History*, *21*(1), 1–24.

Virnig, A., and C. McLeod. 1996. Attitudes toward eating and exercise: A comparison of runners and triathletes. *Journal of Sport Behavior*, *19*(1), 82–91.

Visweswaran, K. 1994. *Fictions of a feminist ethnography*. Minneapolis: University of Minnesota Press.

Ware, J. E., M. Kosinski, and S. D. Keller. 1996. A 12-item short-form health survey: Construction of scales and preliminary tests of reliability and validity. *Med Care, 34,* 220–233.

Yates, A., K. Leehey, and C. M. Shisslak. 1983. Running—an analogue of anorexia? *New England Journal of Medicine*, *308*, 251–255.

Zmijewski, C. F., and M. O. Howard. 2003. Exercise dependence and attitudes toward eating in young adults. *Eating Behaviors, 4*, 181–195.